My Mouth Mirror

(Hate Dental Visits - Take a Peek Through my Mirror!)

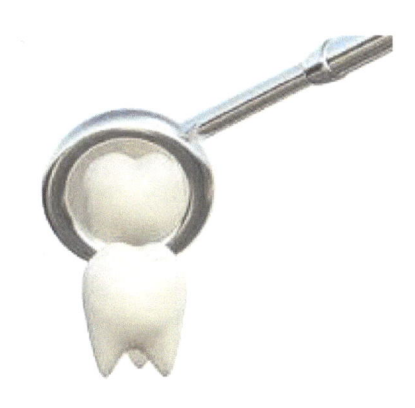

By

Dr. Ajna Abdulrahman

My Mouth Mirror

Introduction

This book was born out of a simple conversation with my older brother, yet that moment changed everything for me. As we discussed dental health, he was struck by the clarity and passion in my explanations. "You should write a book," he said, almost offhandedly, but his words lodged themselves in my mind. I'd never thought of myself as an author.

I'd only ever read dental textbooks or professional material—never something unrelated to my work. But his encouragement stayed with me, sparking an idea that began to feel like both a challenge and a call.

For years, I've been in the habit of writing notes—scribbles about my day, my experiences in dentistry, interesting cases, and reflections I rarely share aloud. Writing has been a kind of therapy, a place where I can untangle my thoughts, document new discoveries, and capture memorable moments in my career. Little did I know that these notes would someday form the foundation of a book.

After nearly a decade in dentistry—starting with my studies bachelor's in dental surgery BDS at Rajiv Gandhi University in India and continuing with my practice and growth in the United Kingdom—I realized I had a wealth of practical insights that could benefit others. I decided to write a simple, approachable book about dental health that anyone could understand whether they're a patient wanting to care for their teeth, a dental professional seeking clarity, or even someone curious about a career in dentistry.

This book, "My Mouth Mirror," offers readers a straightforward journey into the essentials of dental care, drawing from my personal experiences, studies, and encounters over the past eight years. Through these pages, I hope to shine a light on the often-overlooked importance of oral health, to demystify the field of dentistry, and to share my passion for helping others achieve healthier, brighter smiles.

Let this book be your guide to understanding dentistry from the inside out—a look through my very own "Mouth mirror."

Acknowledgements

First and foremost, my deepest gratitude goes to my parents, Mr. CK Abdul Rahman and Mrs. Jameela Abdul Rahman, whose unwavering support and guidance laid the foundation for everything I have achieved.

To my brothers Mr. Big B and Mr. AAR, thank you for always cheering me on and inspiring me to push further. To my older brother, in particular—without your insightful suggestions and the seed you planted in my mind, this book would never have come to life.

To my husband, Naz, whom I eagerly look forward to surprising with this book—you are my rock and my biggest supporter, and I am so grateful for all that you mean to me.

And to my son, Emir Abram—my little one, you are my heart and my hope. I dream that one day, you'll read this book and feel proud of the journey I took.

Also, my heartfelt thank you to Miss Amna Waris, my dear friend and fellow book lover, for her valuable help in tidying up the loose ends.

And all my love on all my beautiful family and friends.

Disclaimer

This book is intended solely for informational purposes, providing basic insights into dentistry. It is not a substitute for professional or expert advice, diagnosis, or treatment. The author and publisher make no representations or warranties regarding the accuracy, completeness, or suitability of the information provided and assume no responsibility for any consequences arising from its use. Every individual's circumstances are unique, and the guidance offered in this book may not be appropriate for your situation. Always seek the advice of qualified professionals for any specific dental or medical concerns. All images used in this book have been captured during practice sessions with permissions or sourced from online learning platforms that do not impose copyright restrictions.

Contents

Introduction v

Acknowledgements vii

Disclaimer ix

1. A Dental Voyage - My Mouth Mirror 2
2. From Fear to Trust 6
3. Behind the Mask – Is Dentist Doctor? 18
4. It's Just a Tooth – The Tired Smiles 25
5. Dental Care for Your Child's Early Years 42
6. Teeth: An Early Warning System for Overall Health 53
7. A Clean Plate for a Clean Meal: Why Your Mouth Deserves the Same Care 64
8. When to Visit the Dentist: A Lifetime of Care for a Lifetime of Smiles 70
9. Shedding And Eruption Timeline 76
10. Oral Cavity - Know Me Well 84
11. Dental Team – A Family 89
12. Do Medical Histories Matter in Dental Care? 95
13. I am Old, and so is My Tooth! 101
14. I Am Your Tooth – What's My Role? 105
15. Miscellaneous Oral Cavity Atlas 108
Epilogue: A Love Affair with Dentistry 121

Chapter 1

A Dental Voyage - My Mouth Mirror

My passion for becoming a doctor began when I was just a child. I would tell everyone, with great conviction, that I would grow up to be a doctor. My inspiration came from our family doctor, a close friend of my father, who treated all of us for general consultations. Every time I saw him interact with patients, I was deeply impressed by his knowledge, the way he cared for others, and the respect he earned from the community. He would often gift me disposable syringes and books, including picture anatomy books and medical encyclopedias, starting when I was just seven years old. I would spend hours pretending to be a doctor, playing with my friends and cousins. As I grew older, my dream of becoming a doctor grew more serious.

At the age of 16, I started preparing for the entrance exams, which were essential to secure a spot in a government medical college back home. Scoring well was crucial, as private colleges were financially out of reach for my family. The journey of preparation through coaching centers was intense, and I had high hopes for a good rank. However, despite my efforts, I didn't qualify for a medical seat in my home state. Instead, I qualified for a dental seat in another state, which left me confused and uncertain.

Dentistry had never been part of my plan, and I knew very little about it. The only thing that kept me going was the knowledge that I would still earn the title of "doctor" after five years of study.

With limited time to explore my options, I leapt and started my dental studies at the university. In the first year, I found comfort in studying many of the same subjects taught in general medicine—particularly anatomy, physiology, and biochemistry— although the focus was mainly on the head and neck. It was during a seminar by a professor from Rajiv Gandhi University on the topic of oral health and its connection to overall body systems that my perspective on dentistry changed entirely. The seminar opened my eyes to the importance of the oral cavity and its links to systemic health.

From that moment, I embraced my path and proudly identified myself as a dental student.

The first year was tough, with challenging subjects and demanding practicals, but I made it through. The second year was even more intense, with subjects like pharmacology, microbiology, pathology, and the addition of dental materials and oral pathology. It was overwhelming, especially with the pressure of seeing seniors struggle to clear their exams for years. Nevertheless, with persistence and continuous hard work, I successfully passed the second year and, soon after, the third and final years, which were filled with even more demanding subjects and practical exams.

My final year was especially challenging, I faced a deeply challenging and unfair situation that tested me both mentally and emotionally. My record books were torn apart by a Periodontics lecturer in college, and my clinical cases were canceled without any clear reason. This experience was part of a broader pattern of bullying that left me feeling mentally exhausted and helpless. As the final theory exams approached, I was given only a few days to redo everything from scratch. The thought of failing my final year, after so much hard work, felt like the end of the world to me at that age. However, instead of giving up, I chose to rise above adversity. I summoned the courage to take on the challenge, determined not to let this situation define my future. I worked tirelessly, completing my records and clinical cases again in record time, all while facing numerous other obstacles. Despite the immense pressure, I persevered and not only passed my final exams but achieved excellent scores. To my immense pride, scoring good marks in all subjects, I emerged as the subject topper in Orthodontics.

This experience taught me the power of resilience, determination, and believing in oneself, even in the face of overwhelming odds. It remains a defining moment in my journey, shaping the person I am today. But through it all, my father was my rock—always encouraging me to stay strong, never to give up, and to face challenges head-on with confidence.

Like many students, I thought that once I completed my degree, I would enter a bright future, ready to help people and become a respected doctor. But the reality was much different. The challenges didn't end with my degree. I quickly realized that there is a common misconception among the public that some don't consider dentists to be "real" doctors, and many believe that dentistry is limited to teeth extractions. These encounters were disheartening, and I felt an urgent need to educate people about the importance of dentistry.

The journey didn't end there. Patients would often come in with fear or express their dislike for dentists, which added to the ongoing struggle. Despite these challenges, I wanted to find a platform to share my experiences, not only for those in the dental field but also to educate patients about the value of what we do.

I am not a professional writer or an experienced author, but through this book, I hope to shed some light on the world of dentistry, my journey, and the importance of oral health.

Chapter 2

From Fear to Trust

One morning, a patient walked in. Before we could even greet each other, she blurted out, "I hate dentists, and I hate coming to the dentist. But here I am, ready to be tortured."

By that point in my career, I had learned to take such comments in stride—objectively, not personally. As healthcare professionals, we're human too, but when faced with a nervous patient, it's important to focus on them, not ourselves. I smiled warmly, gestured for her to sit in the dental chair, and responded, "Well, I'm proud of you, and I really appreciate that even though you hate everything about this, you're still here taking care of your oral health."

I could see her expression softened, and she smiled back at me. She thanked me, and soon enough, she opened up about her fears, sharing the past dental experiences that had left her feeling anxious. I quickly realized that the key to this interaction would be building her trust, assuring her that she was in safe hands and that we were focused on preventive care to protect her health.

We had a meaningful conversation, which set the tone for the session. I took extra precautions, using a numbing gel as a proactive measure. I had sensed from her earlier comments that she was extremely sensitive, and even the thought of touching her gums made her anxious. By numbing her with the gel something I explained and did with her consent—I ensured she didn't have to ask for it or experience any discomfort.

The session went smoothly, much to her relief. Afterwards, the patient unexpectedly burst into tears not from fear or pain, but from joy. She hugged me, saying it was her first positive experience with a dental professional. I couldn't have been happier, and now she's a regular patient.

This experience again assured me: what many patients truly need is empathy.

Taking the time to understand them as individuals, speaking to them as people before assuming the role of a professional, and offering reassurance can turn a dreaded appointment into a positive experience. By building trust and showing care, we can offer not just treatment but comfort and that's often what they value most. I always keep myself ready understanding all basic points why people hate dental visits.

Why people hate dental visits:

Many people dislike or even fear dental visits for a variety of reasons, which can range from psychological factors to physical discomfort. Here are some common reasons why dental visits are often dreaded:

1. **Fear of Pain**

   - Dental procedures like drilling, extractions, or root canals are often associated with pain. Even though modern dentistry uses anesthesia to minimize discomfort, many people still fear the possibility of pain or remember painful past experiences.

2. **Anxiety and Dental Phobia**

   - Some individuals suffer from dental anxiety or dental phobia, which can stem from negative childhood experiences, the fear of losing control, or just general nervousness about the unknown. For some, even the sound of dental tools can trigger anxiety.

3. **Previous Negative Experiences**

   - A bad experience during a past dental visit, such as excessive pain, poor communication from the dentist, or a procedure that went wrong, can create a lasting aversion to future visits.

4. **Fear of Needles and Injections**

   - Many dental procedures involve local anesthesia, which requires injections. Fear of needles is common, and for some, this alone can make them dread going to the dentist.

5. **Cost Concerns**
   - Dental care can be expensive, especially for those without insurance. The cost of treatments like fillings, crowns, and root canals can lead to stress or even avoidance of visits altogether.

6. **Discomfort with the Sensations**

   - Gag reflex, discomfort from lying back for long periods, or the unpleasant feeling of tools in the mouth can be distressing. Some people feel claustrophobic or simply uncomfortable with the physical sensations that come with dental procedures.

7. **Embarrassment About Oral Health**

   - People who haven't seen a dentist in a long time or who have poor oral health may feel embarrassed or ashamed about the condition of their teeth. This fear of being judged by the dentist or staff can make them avoid appointments.

8. **Loss of Control**

   - Lying down with your mouth open while someone else works on your teeth can make some people feel vulnerable and out of control, which contributes to their discomfort.

9. **Invasive Nature of the Procedures**

   - Dental procedures are often viewed as intrusive because they involve working inside a person's mouth, which is an intimate and sensitive part of the body. This can create discomfort or aversion.

10. **Fear of the Unknown**

   - Not knowing what a procedure will entail or fearing that a routine checkup might reveal the need for unexpected treatments can create fear of the unknown, making people reluctant to go.

11. **Sensory Overload**

   - Dental offices are filled with bright lights, loud noises from tools, strong smells, and the feeling of various instruments in the mouth, which can lead to sensory overload for some individuals.

12. **Time Constraints**

   - Busy schedules can make people reluctant to take time off for dental appointments, especially if the appointments require multiple visits or long procedures.

13. **Cultural or Family Influence**

   - Negative attitudes toward dentists can sometimes be passed down from family members or social circles, leading to a general dislike or mistrust of dentists, even if the individual hasn't had a bad personal experience.

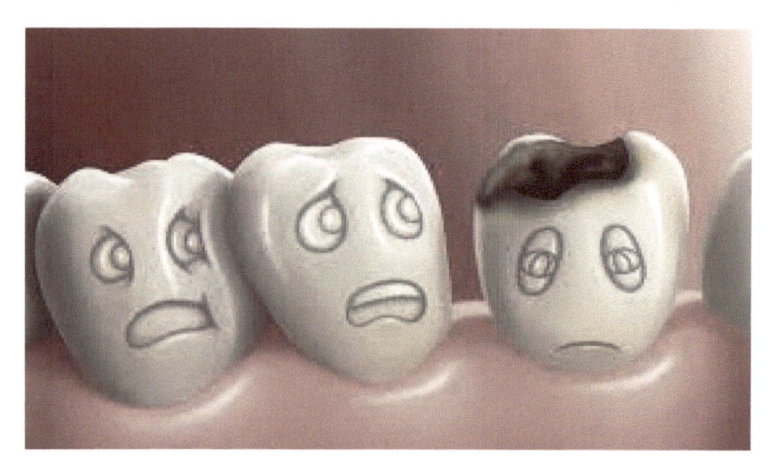

Ways to Address Dental Anxiety:

- Open communication with the dentist about fears and concerns.

- Sedation dentistry options, such as nitrous oxide or oral sedation, for those with significant anxiety.

- Distraction techniques, like listening to music or watching videos during the appointment.

- Choosing a dentist who is experienced in treating anxious patients and offers a calm, understanding approach.

Regular dental visits are important for maintaining oral health, and many dentists are aware of these concerns and are willing to work with patients to make the experience more comfortable.

Creating a positive experience in dentistry to reduce or eliminate patients' fear and anxiety involves addressing both their emotional and physical discomforts. Here are several strategies to help patients have the best possible experience during their dental visits:

1. **Build Trust Through Communication**

   - Explain everything clearly: Before any procedure, explain step by step what will happen in non-technical terms. This helps reduce fear of the unknown and builds trust.
   - Active listening: Make time to listen to the patient's concerns and anxieties. Let them know their feelings are valid, and work together to address their fears.
   - Provide choices: Offering choices like taking breaks, adjusting seating, or deciding on sedation methods can give patients a sense of control over the situation.

2. **Focus on Comfort**

   - Pain management: Use local anesthetics properly and reassure patients that discomfort will be minimized. Always check on their comfort level during procedures.
   - Comfortable environment: Use comfortable chairs, warm blankets, or neck pillows to help relax patients. Noise-canceling headphones, soft lighting, or even calming music can create a soothing atmosphere.

- Pre-emptive numbing: Offer numbing gel before injections or dental work to prevent pain before it starts. In more anxious patients, offer sedation options like nitrous oxide or oral sedatives.

3. **Create a Relaxing Atmosphere**

- Friendly, welcoming staff: Ensure that your staff is warm, empathetic, and trained to address patient fears. First impressions matter, so friendly greetings and reassuring attitudes can make a big difference.
- Office aesthetics: Design a calming, modern office environment with soothing colours, plants, or relaxing artwork. Consider offering entertainment, like TVs on the ceiling for patients to watch during treatment or even relaxing scents like lavender.

4. **Use Technology to Reduce Discomfort**

- Modern tools: Invest in advanced technology that minimizes discomfort. For example, digital X-rays, laser dentistry (which can reduce the need for drilling), or pain-free injections can significantly enhance the patient experience.
- Clear communication through visual aids: Use digital tools like intra-oral cameras or 3D imaging to show patients what's happening with their teeth, so they understand the necessity of treatment and feel more involved.

5. **Offer Flexible Appointment Scheduling**

- Accommodate patient schedules: Provide convenient appointment times, including early morning, evening, or weekend slots, to reduce stress about missing work or school.

- Shorter, efficient visits: Use streamlined processes and technology to reduce the time patients spend in the chair, especially for routine procedures like cleanings.

6. Address Financial Concerns Openly

- Transparent pricing: Offer clear, upfront explanations of treatment costs and options. Patients appreciate knowing what to expect financially and can feel more in control of their treatment plans.
- Flexible payment plans: Consider offering affordable payment options or dental memberships to alleviate financial stress.

7. Offer Sedation Options

- Sedation dentistry: Offer varying levels of sedation, from mild (nitrous oxide or "laughing gas") to more advanced conscious sedation, depending on the patient's level of anxiety. Let patients know that sedation is available if they are nervous.

8. Implement a Personalized Approach

- Know your patients: Ask about their preferences, fears, or past negative experiences, and tailor the treatment approach to each individual.
- Build rapport: Develop relationships over time by engaging with patients personally. Small gestures like remembering personal details or their preferences for how they like to be treated can make a big difference.
- Follow-up: Check-in after major procedures with a follow-up call or message to see how they're feeling. This shows care and builds trust.

9. **Educate Patients on Prevention:**

- Emphasize preventive care: Help patients understand the importance of regular cleanings and checkups to prevent more painful and complex procedures later.

- Encourage them to view dental visits as part of maintaining overall health.

- Provide home-care tips: Teach patients how to maintain their oral hygiene at home to prevent future problems, which can also reduce their anxiety about future visits.

10. **Involve the Patient in Treatment Decisions**

- Offer treatment options: When appropriate, provide patients with different treatment options, explaining the pros and cons of each. This empowers them to make informed choices, reducing fear of the unknown.

- Use visual aids: Showing patients images or videos of what you plan to do (e.g., using intra-oral cameras or models) can make procedures less intimidating and easier to understand.

11. **Minimize Wait Times**

- Timely appointments: Patients often become more anxious when they have to wait. Keep appointments running on time to reduce the period when patients' anxiety can build.

- Create distractions in the waiting area: If wait times are unavoidable, have entertainment options like magazines, TV, or tablets for patients to use while they wait.

12. Implement Relaxation Techniques

- Breathing exercises: Teach patients breathing or relaxation techniques to use before and during their visit. Deep breathing or mindfulness techniques can help calm nerves.

- Distractions during treatment: Provide distractions, such as listening to music, podcasts, or audio books. Some dental offices offer virtual reality headsets for distraction during procedures.

13. Positive Reinforcement

- Celebrate small wins: Acknowledge patients' bravery or progress, especially if they have dental anxiety. Positive reinforcement can help build confidence for future visits.

- Offer rewards: For younger patients or anxious adults, a small reward or token for completing a visit can create positive associations with the experience.

14. Continuing Education for Staff

- Train staff on patient anxiety: Regularly educate your team on how to manage anxious patients and how to make the dental experience less intimidating. Understanding patient psychology is key to improving patient care.

- Ongoing feedback: Implement a system for gathering patient feedback after visits to identify areas of improvement and make necessary adjustments to the patient experience.

By focusing on patient comfort communication and using modern technology, dental visits can become more pleasant and anxiety-free. Making the experience personal, gentle, and transparent helps foster long-term trust and can ultimately make dental care something patients no longer dread.

Chapter 3

Behind the Mask – Is the Dentist Doctor?

Stress is real, and the workplace is often a tough environment. Whether you're a dentist or any other professional, the pressure is undeniable. But for a dentist, it can be particularly challenging when patients are anxious or difficult to manage. The oral cavity, after all, is one of the most sensitive parts of the body. While it's perfectly understandable for patients to feel nervous, especially during their first visit, it's crucial for both the patient and the dentist to find common ground. Clear communication and mutual understanding can make all the difference.

One morning, I was assisting my chief dental surgeon as part of my probation period. A patient came in complaining of severe pain in her lower right back tooth. After examining her, the chief advised her to take medication and return for an X-ray, which would help us make a proper diagnosis and decide on the best course of treatment. He also took the time to explain the treatment plan thoroughly. However, the patient was reluctant. She insisted that medication alone would be enough, claiming that further treatment was too expensive. Moreover, she expressed skepticism about root canal treatments, suggesting that dentists recommend them primarily for financial gain.

Despite my chief's efforts to explain the importance of the treatment, the patient refused to proceed and left with just the medication. Unfortunately, she only took the medication for one day, stopping once the pain subsided. When she returned, she had developed a severe abscess and swelling. We drained the pus and prescribed medication again, but once more, the patient didn't follow through. She neither completed the course of medication nor came in for her next appointment, which eventually led to a serious condition called Ludwig's angina.

Ludwig's angina is a potentially life-threatening bacterial infection that occurs on the floor of the mouth. It can develop after an untreated tooth infection or injury. If not managed aggressively, it can lead to airway obstruction and other critical complications. The patient was rushed to the ICU for emergency treatment.

This experience left a lasting impression on me. I often reflection why situations like this arise—why some patients are reluctant to trust their dentist or fail to take oral health seriously. Over time, I've come to realize that dentistry is far more complex than it appears. It's not just about diagnosing problems and offering solutions; it requires immense effort to build trust and foster clear communication with patients.

As dentists, we invest a lot of energy into helping patients understand the importance of their oral health. But it's not always easy. Sometimes, it takes more than just professional knowledge; it takes patience, empathy, and an ability to connect with patients on a deeper level to achieve the best outcomes.

Many people don't consider dentists as "doctors" in the same way they view physicians, largely due to misunderstandings about the training and role of dentists. This misconception stems from a few key factors, such as differences in education paths, societal views, and the specific nature of dentistry as a medical field. Let's explore these points in detail:

1. **Education and Terminology Differences**

   - Degree Titles: Dentists typically earn a Doctor of Dental Surgery (DDS) or Doctor of Dental Medicine (DMD) degree or Bachelor in Dental Surgery (BDS). All 3 are equivalent and represent the same level of education and clinical training. However, because these degrees don't explicitly say "Doctor of Medicine," some people mistakenly believe dentists aren't "real" doctors.

   - Specialized Focus: Dentistry is a highly specialized field focused on oral health, which is just one aspect of the broader medical world. Because dentists don't treat the whole body in the same way general physicians do, people might overlook their role as doctors.

   - Education Requirements: Dentists undergo rigorous training similar to medical doctors, including four years of undergraduate studies followed by four years of dental school, which mirrors the structure of medical school. They also must complete clinical training and often specialize further through additional residency programs.

2. **Societal Views on Dentistry**

- Perception of Dentistry as Separate: Many people view dentistry as distinct from mainstream medicine because dental clinics are usually separate from hospitals and traditional medical practices. This separation in how dental and medical services are delivered can lead to the belief that dentists are not part of the broader healthcare system.

- Focus on Teeth: Because dentists are seen as "just working on teeth," which many consider less vital compared to organs like the heart or lungs, some underestimate the importance of oral health in overall health. This leads to a narrow view of their role rather than understanding that oral health is integral to general well-being.

- Preventive Care Misunderstanding: Much of what a dentist does involves preventive care, which can be undervalued. People might think of "doctors" as those who intervene during a health crisis, while dentists often focus on preventing problems before they become emergencies.

3. **Cultural Factors**

   - Media Representation: Doctors in television and movies are almost always portrayed as physicians or surgeons, rarely dentists. This reinforces a narrow view of what it means to be a "doctor."
   - Historical Division: Historically, dentistry and medicine were seen as distinct professions, with dentistry evolving separately from general medicine. This division has lingered despite dentists having "doctor" status.

What is a Doctor?

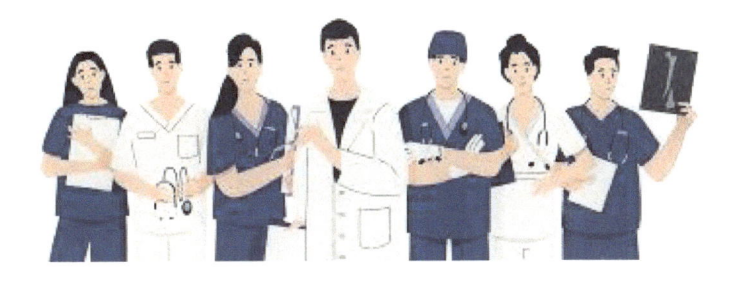

The term "doctor" is broad and can refer to anyone with advanced knowledge and education in a specific field, not just physicians. Here's a breakdown of what it means to be a doctor:

1. **Doctor:**

   - A "doctor" comes from the Latin word docere, meaning "to teach." Traditionally, a doctor is someone with a doctorate-level education, which can be in various fields, including medicine, law, philosophy, and dentistry.

   - Many professions use the title "doctor," such as:

   - Medical doctors (MDs): Focus on general body health.

   - Dentists (DDS/DMDs/BDS): Focus on oral and dental health.

   - PhDs: Focus on research and academics in a particular subject.

   - Chiropractors (DCs): Specialize in musculoskeletal health.

   - Veterinarians (DVMs): Focus on animal health.

2. **Medical Definition:**

   - A doctor, in a healthcare context, is someone licensed to diagnose, treat, and manage medical conditions. Dentists meet this criterion as they diagnose and treat diseases related to the teeth, gums, and mouth.
   - Physicians (MDs or DOs) are general medical doctors who treat the body as a whole, but dentists are specialists in oral health and undergo medical training specific to this field.

3. **Doctor's Role in Society:**

- Healer/Expert: The core role of a doctor is to prevent, diagnose, and treat health issues

No doubt, dentists are doctors, and dental healthcare professionals play a vital role in preventive care, as well as offering a wide range of treatments. In fact, the field of dentistry is even broader, encompassing cosmetic aspects like smile design. After all, who doesn't appreciate a beautiful smile? It's hard to imagine a person without one, and a bad smile can significantly impact confidence. Dentistry not only addresses health concerns but also enhances the aesthetics of a person's smile, which is an integral part of human expression.

Chapter 4

It's Just a Tooth – The Tired Smiles

It was a typical afternoon, though my lunch hadn't been the best, and I was feeling exhausted from a busy day. Despite not being much of a coffee enthusiast, I couldn't resist a second cup. I needed something to jolt my central nervous system and get that adrenaline rush going so I could muster enough energy to engage with my next patient. With the first sip of coffee, I felt the slow, familiar kick of alertness. As I drank, I found myself reflecting on coffee alternatives, especially considering its side effects.

Soon, my afternoon patient arrived. I had gathered my energy and was fully ready to greet him—but it quickly became clear we were complete opposites in that moment. He walked in utterly drained from his workday, barely managing to wish me back. It was amusing to see such a contrast—me, buzzing with caffeine, and him, on the brink of dozing off. He even joked that he might fall asleep during the treatment, which made the situation feel even more surreal. I had the energy for an in-depth conversation, but he was clearly in no mood for one. The irony wasn't lost on me, and I couldn't help but smile at how funny it was to have two people in such different states sharing the same room.

During the exam, I made several observations, but what really caught my attention was his generalized demineralization of enamel. After the session, I felt compelled to bring it up. Despite his fatigue, I wanted to stress the importance of addressing it—dental health is never "just teeth."

When I mentioned my findings, he looked at me, clearly exhausted, and with a tired smile, said, "Do you really want to talk about this? It's just teeth. I'll survive." He laughed, but there was a hint of pity in it. At that moment, I knew I had to tread lightly. I didn't want to overwhelm him, but I also didn't want to let dental neglect slip by unnoticed. So, I kept it brief, giving him a gentle explanation of the condition, then let him go without pushing too hard.

Though I'm proud of myself for handling it tactfully, I couldn't shake the feeling of wanting to help him more. His dismissive attitude towards his oral health made me realize how often people underestimate the importance of their teeth. I genuinely wanted to provide him with the knowledge and support to prevent further damage.

Generalized demineralization of enamel refers to the widespread loss of minerals (such as calcium and phosphate) from the tooth surface, weakening the enamel and making teeth more susceptible to decay. Several factors can contribute to this process:

1. Poor Oral Hygiene:

- Inadequate brushing and flossing allow plaque, a sticky film of bacteria, to build up on teeth. Bacteria in plaque produce acids that erode enamel and lead to demineralization.

2. High Sugar and Acidic Diet:

- Sugary Foods and Drinks: Frequent consumption of sugary foods and beverages (soda, candy, fruit juices) feeds oral bacteria, leading to acid production that breaks down enamel.

- Acidic Foods and Drinks: Consuming acidic foods and drinks (e.g., citrus fruits, soda, energy drinks) directly weakens enamel by lowering the pH in the mouth, initiating the demineralization process.

3. Acidic Saliva (Low pH):

- Dry Mouth (Xerostomia): Saliva neutralizes acids and helps remineralise enamel. Conditions or medications that reduce saliva flow can result in a more acidic environment, leading to demineralization.

- Frequent Snacking: Eating small amounts of food frequently increases acid production, especially when saliva has less time to neutralize the acids between meals.

4. Acid Reflux (Gastroesophageal Reflux Disease - GERD):

- GERD can cause stomach acids to flow back into the mouth, eroding enamel and causing generalized demineralization, especially on the back teeth and the surfaces facing the throat.

5. Frequent Vomiting (Bulimia or Other Conditions):

- Conditions that involve frequent vomiting (e.g., bulimia, morning sickness in pregnancy) expose teeth to stomach acid, leading to significant erosion and demineralization of the enamel, especially on the inner surfaces of teeth.

6. Fluoride Deficiency:

- Fluoride helps to strengthen enamel and resist acid attacks. Inadequate fluoride exposure (e.g., from non-fluoridated water or lack of fluoride toothpaste) can make enamel more vulnerable to demineralization.

7. Malnutrition or Vitamin Deficiencies:

- Vitamin D and Calcium Deficiency: Lack of these nutrients, important for healthy tooth development and maintenance, can weaken enamel and lead to demineralization.

- Poor Diet: A diet lacking in essential nutrients can compromise enamel integrity and make it more prone to acid attacks.

8. Orthodontic Appliances (Braces):

- Poor oral hygiene around braces or other orthodontic appliances can trap food and plaque, leading to localized acid production and demineralization, especially around the brackets.

9. Coeliac Disease:

- Coeliac disease can cause enamel defects and demineralization due to malabsorption of nutrients like calcium and vitamin D, both of which are essential for strong enamel.

10. Medications:

- Acidic Medications: Some medications, such as certain cough syrups or chewable vitamins, are acidic and can contribute to enamel erosion.
- Medications Causing Dry Mouth: Drugs like

antihistamines, antidepressants, and those used for high blood pressure can reduce saliva production, increasing the risk of demineralization.

11. Genetic Disorders (e.g., Amelogenesis Imperfecta):

- This rare genetic condition affects enamel formation, leading to weak, poorly mineralized enamel that is prone to demineralization and erosion.

12. Bruxism (Teeth Grinding):

- Grinding or clenching teeth (bruxism), especially at night, can wear down the enamel, making it more susceptible to demineralization.

13. Exposure to Environmental Acids:

- Chlorinated Swimming Pools: Prolonged exposure to improperly chlorinated pool water, which is often acidic, can lead to enamel demineralization in swimmers.

- Workplace Exposure: Workers in certain environments (e.g., battery factories or those exposed to acidic fumes) may be exposed to acids that can erode enamel.

14. Systemic Conditions (e.g., Diabetes):

- Conditions like diabetes, which can lead to changes in saliva composition and increase susceptibility to infection, may also contribute to demineralization by promoting a more acidic oral environment.

15. Frequent Use of Whitening Products:

- Overuse of highly acidic tooth-whitening products can weaken enamel and promote demineralization, especially if used improperly.

Prevention and Remineralization Strategies:

- Use fluoride toothpaste to strengthen enamel.

- Limit intake of sugary and acidic foods/drinks.

- Practice good oral hygiene by brushing and flossing regularly.

- Drink plenty of water to promote saliva production.

- Get regular dental check-ups to catch early signs of demineralization and receive professional fluoride treatments or sealants.

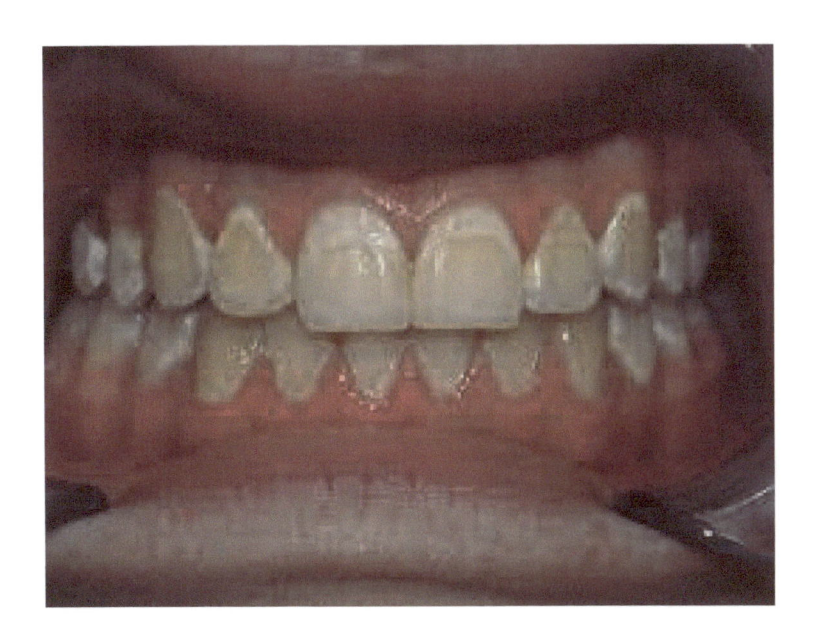

Addressing the underlying causes and maintaining proper oral care can help prevent or reverse early demineralization of enamel.

Certain systemic conditions and diseases can manifest signs and symptoms in the teeth or oral cavity. Some of these signs may indicate an underlying health issue. Here are key signs that suggest a tooth problem may be related to systemic conditions or diseases:

1. Gum Disease (Periodontal Disease) and Systemic Health:

 - Diabetes: Uncontrolled diabetes can lead to more severe gum disease, resulting in bleeding, swollen, and receding gums.
 - Heart Disease: Chronic periodontal disease has been linked to cardiovascular conditions, and severe gum infections may indicate an increased risk of heart disease or stroke.
 - Osteoporosis: Bone loss in the jaw, leading to tooth loss, can be related to osteoporosis.

2. Erosion and Decay:

 - Gastroesophageal Reflux Disease (GERD): Acid reflux

can cause stomach acid to erode the enamel of the teeth, leading to thinning and sensitivity.

- Eating Disorders (Bulimia): Repeated vomiting exposes teeth to stomach acids, causing severe enamel erosion and tooth decay.

3. Tooth and Jaw Pain:

- Sinus Infections: Pain in the upper teeth, especially the molars, can sometimes be related to sinus infections, as the roots of these teeth are close to the sinus cavities.

- Temporomandibular Joint Disorders (TMD): Chronic jaw pain or clicking can be related to systemic conditions like arthritis or fibromyalgia.

4. Delayed or Abnormal Tooth Development:

- Vitamin Deficiencies: Vitamin D or calcium deficiency can lead to poor tooth formation, delayed eruption, or soft, weakened enamel.

- Genetic Disorders (e.g., Amelogenesis Imperfecta): This can result in discolored, soft, or malformed teeth, indicating a genetic condition affecting enamel formation.

5. Mouth Ulcers and Lesions:

- Autoimmune Diseases (e.g., Lupus, Crohn's Disease): Recurring mouth ulcers or lesions can be a sign of an autoimmune condition affecting the mucous membranes.

-Oral Cancer: Persistent sores or lesions in the mouth that don't heal may indicate oral cancer, which can be associated with systemic conditions like HPV or immune suppression.

6. Dry Mouth (Xerostomia):

- Sjogren's Syndrome: This autoimmune disease affects the salivary glands, leading to dry mouth, which increases the risk of cavities and oral infections.

- Medications or Chemotherapy: Some systemic treatments for conditions like cancer or hypertension can lead to reduced saliva production, causing dry mouth.

7. Tooth Loss:

- HIV/AIDS: Advanced HIV can cause oral issues like severe periodontal disease, which may lead to tooth loss or infections.

- Nutritional Deficiencies: Deficiencies in calcium, vitamin C, or vitamin D can contribute to weakened tooth structure and loss of teeth.

8. Discoloration or Staining:

- Fluorosis: Excess fluoride intake during tooth development can cause white or brown spots on teeth.

- Jaundice (Liver Disease): Yellowing of the teeth and gums may indicate liver problems, as bilirubin buildup can cause a yellowish tinge to the mucous membranes.

These signs suggest that oral health and systemic health are closely connected, and dental symptoms could be early indicators of underlying systemic conditions. Regular dental check-ups can help identify these issues early on.

In children, the condition of the teeth and oral cavity can also provide signs of underlying systemic diseases or the side effects of medications. Here are some key signs to watch for that may indicate systemic conditions or medication side effects:

1. Delayed or Abnormal Tooth Development:

- Nutritional Deficiencies: Lack of essential nutrients (vitamin D, calcium) can lead to delayed tooth eruption, poor enamel formation, or malformed teeth in children.

- Genetic Disorders (e.g., Down Syndrome, Ectodermal Dysplasia): These conditions can cause delayed or abnormal tooth eruption, missing teeth (hypodontia), or improperly formed teeth.

2. Tooth Erosion:

- Gastroesophageal Reflux Disease (GERD): Recurrent acid reflux in children can erode tooth enamel, especially on the back teeth, leading to thinning and sensitivity.

- Eating Disorders (Bulimia, though less common in young children): Repeated vomiting can lead to severe enamel erosion.

3. Increased Tooth Decay (Cavities)

- Diabetes: Children with undiagnosed or poorly controlled diabetes may experience higher rates of tooth decay due to dry mouth (xerostomia) and higher glucose levels in saliva.

- Medications: Certain medications (like antihistamines, asthma inhalers, or those for ADHD) can reduce saliva flow, causing dry mouth, which increases the risk of cavities.

4. Tooth Discoloration:

- Jaundice or Liver Disease: In infants, jaundice or liver disease can lead to yellowing of the teeth or gums.

- Medications (Tetracycline): If tetracycline antibiotics are given to a child under 8 years old or to a mother during pregnancy, it can cause permanent grey, brown, or yellow discolouration of the child's teeth.

- Fluorosis: Overexposure to fluoride during tooth development can cause white or brown streaks on the teeth (fluorosis).

5. Oral Ulcers and Lesions:

- Autoimmune Diseases (e.g., Juvenile Idiopathic Arthritis or Crohn's Disease): Children with autoimmune conditions may develop recurrent ulcers, sores, or inflammation in the mouth.

- Side Effects of Medications: Certain chemotherapy drugs or medications used for epilepsy, like phenytoin, can cause mouth sores or swollen gums (gingival hyperplasia).

6. Gum Disease (Periodontal Disease):

- Diabetes: Children with uncontrolled diabetes may show signs of periodontal disease, including red, swollen, or bleeding gums.
- Leukemia: Unexplained bleeding, swollen gums, or persistent infections can sometimes be early signs of leukemia in children.

7. Tooth and Jaw Pain:

- Sinus Infections: In children, a sinus infection can cause discomfort or pain in the upper teeth.
- Temporomandibular Joint Disorders (TMD): Although less common in young children, TMD can result from systemic conditions like juvenile arthritis, causing jaw pain or difficulty chewing.

8. Tooth Loss or Early Tooth Eruption:

- Hyperthyroidism: This condition can lead to early tooth eruption or loss, along with other symptoms like weight loss or restlessness.

- Malnutrition or Chronic Illness: Systemic illnesses or poor nutrition can lead to premature loss of baby teeth due to weakened tooth structure or poor gum health.

9. Dry Mouth (Xerostomia):

- Side Effects of Medications: Many medications commonly prescribed to children, such as those for asthma, allergies, or ADHD, can reduce saliva production, causing dry mouth. This can lead to an increased risk of cavities and gum disease.

- Cystic Fibrosis: Children with cystic fibrosis often experience thick saliva or dry mouth, increasing the risk of tooth decay.

10. Gingival Overgrowth:

- Side Effects of Medications (e.g., Phenytoin for Seizures): Some seizure medications cause gingival hyperplasia (overgrowth of the gum tissue), which can lead to discomfort and make oral hygiene difficult.

11. Enamel Hypoplasia:

- Nutritional Deficiencies or Systemic Diseases: Conditions

like rickets, which are caused by vitamin D deficiency, can lead to defects in enamel development (enamel hypoplasia), causing weak, pitted, or discolored teeth.

- Congenital Syphilis: Children born with congenital syphilis may have deformed or poorly developed teeth (Hutchinson's teeth), which appear notched or peg-shaped.

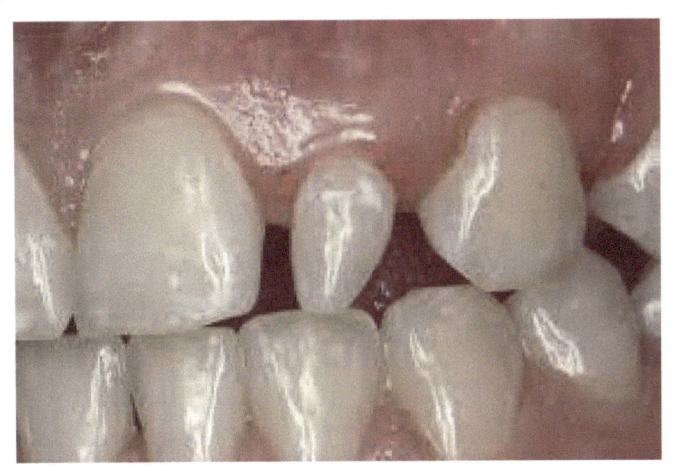

12. Mouth Ulcers or Bleeding:

- Blood Disorders (e.g., Hemophilia or Leukemia): Unexplained or excessive bleeding in the gums, especially during brushing, may indicate a systemic blood disorder.

- Side Effects of Chemotherapy: Cancer treatments like chemotherapy can result in mouth sores, gum bleeding, and other oral health complications.

13. Increased Tooth Sensitivity:

- Coeliac Disease: In some cases, coeliac disease in

children may cause defects in enamel formation, leading to increased sensitivity and discomfort, especially when eating hot or cold foods.

In children, these signs should prompt further investigation to ensure that any underlying systemic health issues or medication side effects are properly addressed. Regular dental check-ups and discussions with pediatricians are essential for monitoring these conditions.

Chapter 5

Dental Care for Your Child's Early Years

"He's just 4 years old; we didn't think he needed a dental visit," one parent explained as they brought their young child to the clinic due to severe tooth pain. They wanted only a quick solution to ease the discomfort, not a right treatment plan.

Upon examination, I was deeply concerned. The child was experiencing severe decay, and the posterior teeth were having Chronic furcal caries. Also the child was having "nursing bottle caries" or "rampant caries." Most of his back teeth had extensive cavities, and many were reduced to root stumps. I felt it was crucial to discuss his condition with his parents and emphasize the importance of early and consistent dental care.

I explained that without proper intervention, his dental issues could lead to long-term problems, including improper eruption of permanent teeth. Since many of his baby teeth had deteriorated to root stumps, they might not fall out naturally. If these decayed teeth were not removed, there was a strong possibility that his adult teeth would erupt misaligned, leading to crowded or crooked teeth.

The parents listened carefully as I outlined a treatment plan and encouraged them to monitor their child's dental development, particularly the stages of shedding baby teeth and the eruption of permanent teeth. They appreciated learning about the timelines for these developmental milestones and were eager to prevent similar issues in the future.

Why Early Dental Care Matters:

It's common for parents to wonder why young children need such diligent dental care. But in reality, dental health begins at birth. By taking a few simple, proactive steps, parents can set the foundation for a lifetime of healthy teeth:

1. **Start Early with Gum Care:**

After each feeding, wipe your newborn's gums with a damp, clean cotton pad. This gentle cleaning helps remove any milk residue, preventing the buildup of lactose on the gums, which can lead to early decay.

2. **Introduce Brushing with the First Tooth:**

Once your baby's teeth begin to emerge, brushing becomes essential to prevent cavities. Use a soft, baby-sized toothbrush and a tiny smear of fluoride toothpaste to gently brush twice daily.

3. Monitor Fluoride Intake:

Check the fluoride level in your local water. If fluoride levels are high, consult your dentist to avoid potential fluorosis, a condition that can cause discoloration and pitting of teeth.

4. Be Mindful of Medications During Breastfeeding:

Breastfeeding mothers should be cautious about any medications they take, as certain medications can affect a baby's dental development, leading to potential staining or structural issues.

5. Schedule Baby's First Dental Visit by 6 Months:

Early dental visits—beginning at 6 months—allow the dentist to check gum health, monitor frenal attachments (which, if too high, can cause spacing between teeth), and assess for any early developmental concerns. Regular visits help create a proactive plan for maintaining a healthy oral environment.

Picture below shows the high frenal attachment also leading to spacing after teeth erupted this is treatable once early diagnosed:

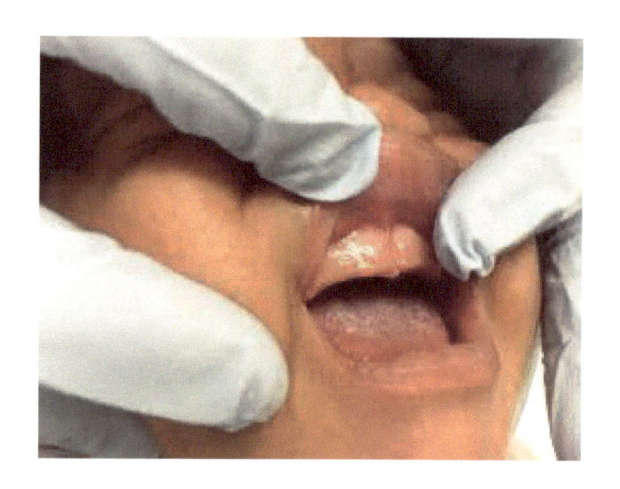

High frenal attachment and Midline Diastema

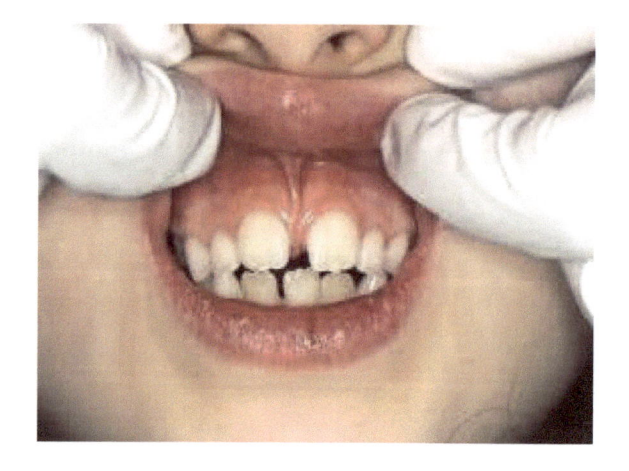

6. Observe Your Child's Sleep and Breathing Patterns:

Keep an eye on your child's sleeping posture and breathing habits. Mouth breathing, for instance, can lead to forward-protruding teeth over time, so it's essential to consult with a dentist or pediatrician if you notice this habit.

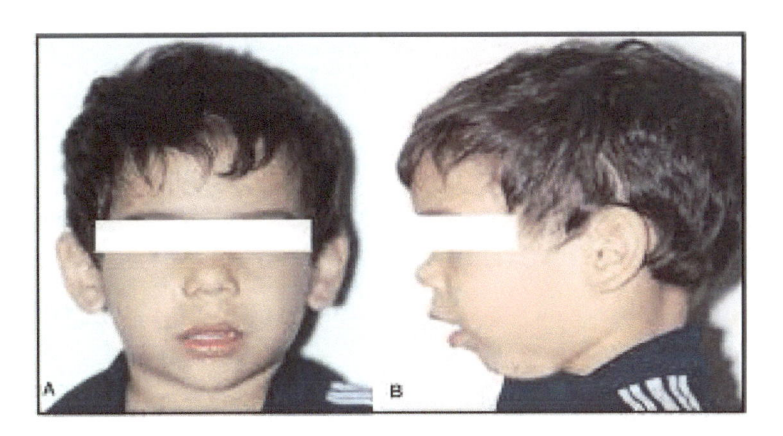

Starting dental care from infancy sets the stage for a lifetime of healthy smiles. Educating yourself on the basics of infant dental care and prioritizing regular check-ups can make a significant difference, not just for your child's current health but also for their future well-being.

Importance of Early Dental Care for Children:

1. Prevention of Early Tooth Decay

• Cleaning a baby's gums and teeth from birth prevents the buildup of bacteria that leads to tooth decay.

• Decay in baby teeth can cause pain infections and impact the child's nutrition and overall health.

2. Foundation for Healthy Adult Teeth

• Baby teeth act as placeholders for adult teeth, helping them come in correctly.

• Early decay or tooth loss can lead to alignment issues in permanent teeth, causing crowding or gaps.

3. Avoidance of Pain and Infections

• Dental infections can be painful and disruptive for children, impacting their ability to eat, sleep, and concentrate.

• Untreated infections in baby teeth can spread to other areas, potentially leading to more serious health issues. Picture below shows how Dental Abscess look like in child:

Dental Abscess and Teeth Decay:

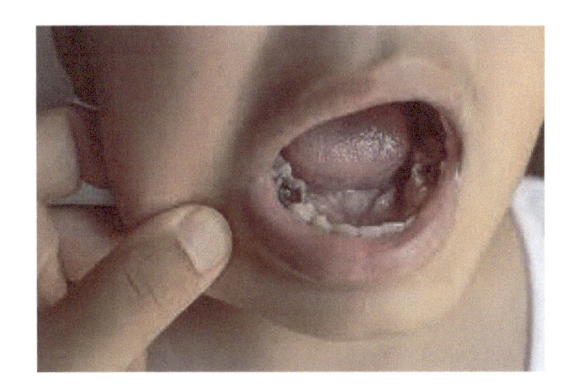

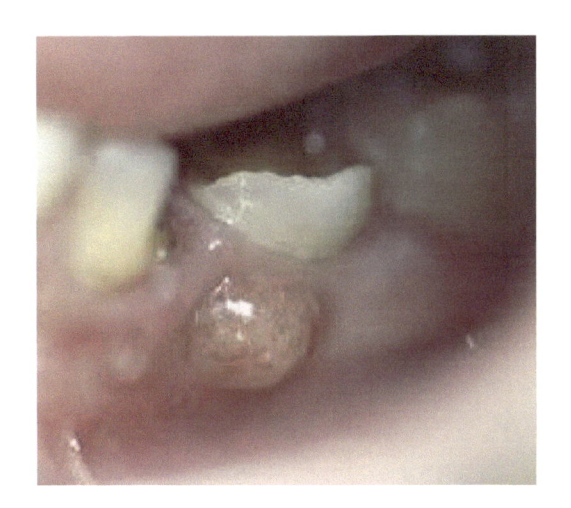

4. **Supporting Speech and Development**

- Healthy teeth play a critical role in the development of speech and articulation.

- Early dental issues can affect a child's ability to speak clearly, which could impact their confidence and communication skills.

5. **Building Good Habits from the Start**

- Introducing brushing and regular check-ups early helps children develop positive oral hygiene habits.

- Familiarity with dental care routines reduces anxiety and encourages lifelong habits for a healthy smile.

- Introducing good brushing technique that should take 2 minutes. Divide the mouth into 6 sections and take 20 seconds to brush each. Then to start with outer surfaces of the lower jaw, then the inner and then the biting surfaces and to repeat with upper jaw. Always using small circular movements near the gumline is most effective.

6. **Monitoring for Developmental Concerns**

- Early dental visits allow professionals to monitor gum health, tooth eruption, frenal attachments (for gaps), and other growth aspects.

- Dentists can identify and address developmental issues such as crowded teeth, mouth breathing, or high frenal attachments early on.

7. **Avoiding Expensive Treatments Later On**

- Addressing minor issues early prevents them from

becoming severe, potentially saving costs and reducing the need for more extensive treatments later.

- Proper care of baby teeth minimizes the chances of complex orthodontic work as the child grows.

8. Protecting General Health

- Poor dental health has been linked to other health conditions, including heart issues and diabetes.

- Early dental care contributes to a strong immune system and overall well-being, as a healthy mouth reduces the risk of infections spreading.

9. Fluoride Exposure and Safety

- Monitoring fluoride exposure early helps prevent both fluorosis (excessive fluoride) and decay (from too little fluoride).

- Ensuring the right fluoride level in water and toothpaste protects teeth from decay while avoiding staining.

10. Awareness of Medication Effects (for Breastfeeding Mothers)

- Medications taken by breastfeeding mothers can affect a baby's developing teeth, potentially leading to staining or structural issues.

- Educating parents on the impact of certain medications helps prevent potential side effects in the child's dental development.

11. Preventing Habit-Related Issues (Thumb-Sucking and Mouth Breathing)

• Early visits allow dentists to advise parents on harmful habits like thumb-sucking, which can affect teeth alignment and jaw development.

• Mouth breathing, if identified early, can be managed to prevent it from causing protruding teeth or jaw misalignment.

12. Creating Positive Dental Experiences

• Regular early visits help children become comfortable with the dental office environment, reducing anxiety.

• Positive dental experiences can create a more cooperative and pleasant experience for children and parents as they grow.

13. Improving Confidence and Social Comfort

• Good oral health contributes to a child's confidence and self-esteem, as children with healthy smiles are more likely to feel comfortable and happy in social settings.

14. Ensuring Proper Nutrition

• Dental pain or decay can interfere with a child's ability to eat a balanced diet, affecting their nutrition and growth.

• Strong, healthy teeth enable children to chew and eat well, supporting their physical development and energy levels.

15. Early Awareness of Eruption and Shedding Timelines

• Parents become aware of when baby teeth should fall out, and permanent teeth should erupt, helping them monitor any irregularities.

- Dentists can guide parents on expected changes, so they're prepared for each stage of dental development.

Understanding these points, parents can see the broad and lasting impact early dental care has on their child's health, confidence, and future well-being.

Chapter 6

Teeth: An Early Warning System for Overall Health

Once a Friday, my third patient of the day entered the clinic with a polite greeting. Yet, beneath his courtesy, he looked noticeably fatigued and somewhat disheartened.

After he settled into the dental chair, he initiated the conversation, explaining his frustrations with oral care. Despite being diligent with brushing, he said, his gums were no healthier, his teeth showed signs of decay, and he'd noticed substantial tartar build-up.

As he spoke, I listened carefully, offering him my full attention. I assured him that I would perform a thorough examination, understanding the importance of addressing both his concerns and any underlying issues.

After examining his teeth and gums, I noted that his oral hygiene practices were exemplary. His frequency of dental visits, technique, and hygiene routines all aligned with best practices. This raised a red flag, as his oral health concerns were not related with his oral care. I then asked him about his sleep patterns, stress levels, and dietary habits—factors that often impact oral health but are frequently overlooked.

During our conversation, he revealed that he had been under significant stress for the past few months and had been struggling with sleep deprivation. I took the opportunity to explain that oral health is not always solely a matter of brushing and flossing. Even when we follow excellent hygiene practices, our teeth, gums, and soft tissues can reveal signs of systemic issues, such as chronic stress, sleep disorders, or other underlying health conditions. These factors can manifest in the mouth as inflammation, gum disease, increased tartar build-up, and even decay.

I advised him to consult with his general physician for a comprehensive blood test and to discuss his stress and sleep concerns. Addressing these factors, I explained, might improve his oral health, as well as his overall well-being.

This case underscores a common misconception: many people believe that if they are meticulous with oral hygiene, they shouldn't experience dental issues. However, our teeth and gums are often a reflection of our body's internal state. Bad breath, tartar build-up, gum problems, and even cavities can signal broader health concerns, sometimes unrelated to dental care itself.

For this reason, it is essential to consider our teeth as an early warning system for systemic conditions. Regular dental visits allow dental professionals to identify these signs early and, when necessary, refer patients to appropriate specialists. Recognizing this link between oral health and overall wellness is vital for both patients and providers, as it reinforces the value of a holistic approach to health care.

Teeth and oral health can indeed act as early indicators of several systemic health conditions. Here are some examples where dental issues might reveal underlying health concerns:

1. **Diabetes**

• Signs in Teeth and Gums: People with diabetes often experience more frequent gum infections (gingivitis and periodontitis) and dry mouth, which can lead to decay and infections.

• Why: High blood sugar can weaken the immune system, making it harder for the body to fight off infections, especially in the gums.

2. **Heart Disease**

• Signs in Teeth and Gums: Chronic gum disease, or periodontitis, has been linked to heart disease. People with inflamed gums may be at a higher risk of cardiovascular problems.

• Why: Inflammation from gum disease can spread through the bloodstream, potentially contributing to plaque build-up in arteries, which is a risk factor for heart disease.

3. **Osteoporosis**

• Signs in Teeth and Jawbone: Osteoporosis can cause a loss of bone density in the jawbone, which may lead to loose teeth, gum recession, and denture instability.

- Why: Since osteoporosis weakens bones, it can also weaken the structures that support the teeth, leading to tooth loss or increased tooth mobility.

4. Gastroesophageal Reflux Disease (GERD)

- Signs in Teeth: GERD can cause enamel erosion, particularly on the inside surfaces of the back teeth.
- Why: Acid from the stomach can flow back into the mouth, wearing down tooth enamel and increasing the risk of decay.

5. Anemia

- Signs in Gums and Mouth: Pale gums, a swollen tongue (glossitis), or sores in the mouth may indicate anemia.
- Why: Low red blood cell counts reduce oxygen flow to body tissues, including the gums and tongue, leading to paleness or other symptoms in the mouth.

6. Eating Disorders (e.g., Bulimia)

- Signs in Teeth: Repeated vomiting introduces stomach acid to the mouth, eroding tooth enamel, especially on the back of the teeth.
- Why: Acid erosion from frequent exposure to stomach acid is a hallmark of bulimia and can lead to significant tooth decay.

7. Vitamin and Nutritional Deficiencies

- Signs in Gums, Tongue, and Teeth: Deficiencies in

vitamins such as vitamin C (linked to bleeding gums and scurvy) and vitamin D (associated with bone and tooth health) can show up in oral health. Lack of B vitamins may also cause sores or inflammation in the mouth.

• Why: Nutritional deficiencies weaken the body's tissues, including the gums and oral soft tissues, leading to symptoms in the mouth.

8. **Autoimmune Disorders (e.g., Sjogren's Syndrome, Lupus)**

• Signs in Saliva Production and Gums: Autoimmune diseases can lead to dry mouth (xerostomia), which increases the risk of decay, gum disease, and oral infections.

• Why: Autoimmune disorders can impair salivary gland function or lead to inflammation in oral tissues.

9. **HIV/AIDS**

• Signs in Gums, Tongue, and Mouth Tissues: Oral signs like persistent mouth ulcers, white lesions (thrush or hairy leukoplakia), and gum disease may be early signs of HIV.

• Why: A weakened immune system from HIV makes it difficult to fend off oral infections, allowing opportunistic infections to flourish.

10. **Chronic Kidney Disease**

• Signs in Breath and Gums: Ammonia-like breath (due to uremia) and gum inflammation are sometimes early signs of kidney issues.

- Why: Kidneys filter waste from the body, and when they aren't functioning properly, waste build-up can cause a range of symptoms, including bad breath and oral changes.

If you notice any persistent or unusual dental or oral health changes, it's a good idea to consult both a dentist and a general healthcare provider. Oral health is often directly linked to overall wellness, and early detection through dental signs can make a significant difference in managing underlying health conditions.

Likewise, stress and sleep issues can have significant effects on oral health as well. Here are some examples:

1. **Bruxism (Teeth Grinding)**

• Signs in Teeth: Teeth grinding, or bruxism, often occurs during sleep and can lead to worn-down teeth, cracks, jaw pain, and even broken dental work.

• Connection to Stress and Sleep: Bruxism is commonly triggered by stress and anxiety. It can also be a sign of sleep disorders, such as sleep apnoea, where teeth grinding occurs as the body struggles to maintain airflow during sleep.

2. **Temporomandibular Joint Disorders (TMD)**

• Signs in Jaw and Face: TMD involves pain or discomfort in the jaw joint, leading to symptoms like jaw clicking, headaches, earaches, and facial pain.

• Connection to Stress: Stress often causes people to clench their jaw unconsciously, especially during sleep, which can strain the temporomandibular joint and lead to TMD.

3. **Dry Mouth (Xerostomia)**

• Signs in Mouth and Gums: Dry mouth can lead to gum inflammation, increased risk of tooth decay, and bad breath.

• Connection to Stress and Sleep: High-stress levels and

anxiety can reduce saliva production, leading to dry mouth. Additionally, some medications prescribed for stress, anxiety, and sleep disorders can cause dry mouth as a side effect.

4. Canker Sores (Aphthous Ulcers)

• Signs in Mouth: Canker sores are small, painful ulcers that appear on the inside of the mouth, cheeks, or gums.

• Connection to Stress: Stress and lack of sleep can weaken the immune system, making people more prone to canker sores. Stress can also disrupt the body's ability to heal, causing these sores to last longer.

5. Gum Disease (Gingivitis and Periodontitis)

• Signs in Gums: Chronic stress can make gum tissues more vulnerable to inflammation and infection, leading to gingivitis (early gum disease) and periodontitis (advanced gum disease).

• Connection to Stress: Stress can lower immunity, which can impair the body's response to oral bacteria, allowing gum disease to develop or worsen. People under stress may also neglect oral hygiene routines or engage in habits like smoking, further increasing their risk.

6. Oral Lichen Planus

• Signs in Mouth: Oral lichen planus appears as white, lace-like patches or sores in the mouth.

• Connection to Stress: While the exact cause is unknown,

stress and anxiety are believed to trigger or worsen Oral lichen planus in susceptible individuals.

7. Burning Mouth Syndrome

- Signs in Mouth: This condition causes a burning sensation in the mouth, often on the tongue, lips, or roof of the mouth, without an identifiable cause.

- Connection to Stress and Sleep: Burning mouth syndrome is often associated with high stress, anxiety or depression it is also more common in people who have disrupted sleep, which may worsen the perception of pain.

8. Sleep Apnoea

- Signs in Teeth and Mouth: People with sleep apnoea may have signs like a scalloped tongue (indentations on the sides from pressing against the teeth) or signs of bruxism (teeth grinding).

- Connection to Sleep: Sleep apnoea is a sleep disorder that causes breathing interruptions during sleep, leading to poor sleep quality and often triggering bruxism as the body struggles to keep the airway open.

9. Weakened Immune Response Leading to Increased Infections

- Signs in Gums and Mouth: Frequent or recurrent infections, such as gum infections or fungal infections (thrush) can be a sign of stress-related immune suppression.

- Connection to Stress and Sleep: Chronic stress and sleep deprivation can weaken the immune system, making the mouth more susceptible to infections that wouldn't typically be a problem when the body is well-rested and less stressed.

In addition to these conditions, lifestyle factors tied to stress like poor diet, smoking, and excessive caffeine or alcohol intake can also contribute to oral health issues. Addressing stress and improving sleep quality can go a long way in promoting both oral and overall health.

Chapter 7

A Clean Plate for a Clean Meal: Why Your Mouth Deserves the Same Care

A patient came in with concerns about bad breath. She told me, "I brush every day, but people still say my breath isn't fresh." I asked if she had ever had a professional dental cleaning, and she admitted she hadn't. In fact, she was fearful of it, believing that scaling could harm her teeth. She believed the hardened calculus deposits on her teeth were part of her natural tooth structure.

For a dental professional, this scenario is quite common. I started by explaining the basics what calculus and plaque are, which is a sticky colorless biofilm of bacteria that forms on the surfaces of teeth. When plaque isn't removed through regular brushing and flossing, it hardens into calculus (tartar), which can turn brown or yellow and cling tightly to the teeth. Tartar can lead to gum inflammation, bleeding, loose teeth, and even severe infections if left untreated.

To illustrate and make her understandable I asked her to imagine eating from a plate that hadn't been washed or traveling in a dirty, unmaintained car. Just as we make sure to wash our plates, maintain our cars, and always prefer to eat nutritious, clean food, our mouths deserve the same attention as we can't imagine eating spoiled food. Infact its almost similar to eating a spoiled food as keeping food deposits in our inter dental spaces for long time and not being aware how bad bacterial build up it causes not just leading to decaying teeth causes issues to gut health. Infact its always high chances of growing yeast or fungi or viruses etc. and we eat with same mouth everyday and in most cases affecting internal system.

We can't expect a clean, healthy experience if our oral hygiene is neglected. An unclean mouth—plagued by unremoved tartar and soft plaque—can lead to bad breath, gum issues, and a host of dental problems.

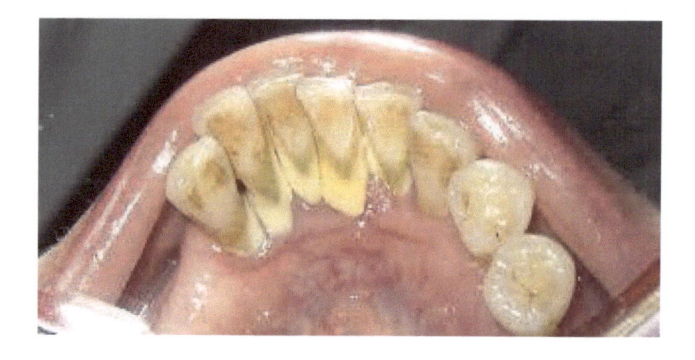

Our mouths are home to beautiful, pearl-like teeth and a sensitive tongue equipped with taste buds. Brushing twice daily and visiting a dental professional every six months are essential steps to ensure a clean, healthy oral environment.

A dental hygiene visit isn't just about "cleaning your teeth." It's a critical part of preventive care that supports your oral and systemic health.

Importance of Oral Hygiene:

The structures in the oral cavity are vulnerable to plaque (a sticky film of bacteria), which can lead to tooth decay, gum disease, and bad breath if not removed regularly. Practicing good oral hygiene is essential for a healthy mouth, which in turn supports overall health. Some key practices include:

- Brushing twice daily to remove plaque and food particles.

- Scraping tongue, which is as important to remove plaque in tongue which is also major source of bacterial build up. Not scraping tongue also leads to condition called "Coated Tongue" without treatment this gunk of bacteria leads to gum disease also can spread infection to body parts. Coated tongues also serious cause of an underlying illness or Leukoplakia a pre-cancerous condition.

- Flossing daily to clean between teeth and below the gum line.

- Rinsing with mouthwash to reduce bacteria.

- Regular dental check-ups every six months to monitor and maintain oral health.

Why a Hygiene Visit is Essential and What to Expect:

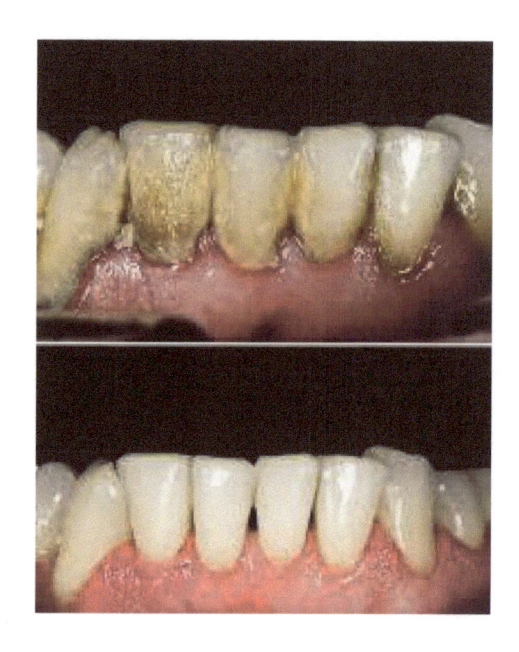

A professional hygiene visit involves much more than just brushing and flossing at home. Here are some key reasons why it's essential:

1. Tartar and Plaque Removal: No matter how well we brush, plaque can still form in hard-to-reach areas, eventually hardening into tartar. Dental hygienists use specialized tools to remove this build-up, especially in areas a toothbrush can't reach.

2. Gum Health Assessment: Hygienists check for signs of gum disease, such as swelling, redness, and bleeding, which

might otherwise go unnoticed. Regular visits help prevent gum disease from advancing.

3. Deep Cleaning: Hygienists perform scaling and polishing to remove plaque and tartar both above and below the gum line (subgingival cleaning). This includes cleaning periodontal pockets, which are gaps that form around the teeth when gums pull away due to inflammation or infection.

4. Prevention of Bad Breath: Tartar and bacteria are major contributors to bad breath. By removing these, a hygiene visit can help eliminate sources of persistent bad odor.

5. Detection of Early Oral Health Issues: Hygienists can spot signs of potential issues, such as early tooth decay, enamel wear, or changes in soft tissue. Detecting these early can prevent more extensive treatments down the line.

6. Inter-dental and Subgingival Care: Hygienists clean between teeth (inter-dental areas) and below the gum line, removing plaque and tartar from areas often missed in routine brushing and flossing.

7. Personalized Oral Health Advice: Hygienists can offer personalized recommendations on brushing, flossing, and products best suited for your specific oral health needs.

8. Long-Term Dental Health: Regular cleanings help maintain the integrity of your teeth and gums over time, reducing the need for more complex and costly dental treatments in the future.

Hygienists are essential partners in your oral health journey, ensuring that every part of your mouth is properly cared for and protected. With their expertise and preventive approach, they play a crucial role in maintaining not only the appearance but also the overall health of your smile.

So, remember, just as you wouldn't eat from a dirty plate, don't let your mouth become neglected. A regular visit to the dental hygienist will keep your teeth, gums, and breath in their best possible condition—clean, fresh, and healthy.

Chapter 8

When to Visit the Dentist: A Lifetime of Care for a Lifetime of Smiles

"My biggest regret," my patient said with a wistful smile, "is that no one told me how important my teeth would be as I got older. If only I'd known when I was young—maybe I'd still have some of my own teeth left for a beautiful smile in my seventies. But here I am with dentures already."

He paused, adjusting his artificial denture. "Growing up, we were told that there was no point in worrying about teeth because we'd lose them anyway once we got older. Now, in my early seventies, I have only my lower teeth left; all my upper teeth are gone. Losing them was painful—much more painful than I'd ever imagined."

"I remember we had a 'Happy Smile Club' at school back in

the 1960s. Dentists seemed like butchers to us back then. Everything about it was scary, and we didn't have a real awareness of oral health or the difference that early care can make. Today, I'd tell the younger generation: start visiting the dentist as soon as your first tooth appears.

Those teeth are precious—more precious than we realize. Your smile, your speech, your ability to eat, to express joy, sadness, love…life itself begins with a healthy smile."

This patient's reflection captures a message that is both heartfelt and essential: dental care isn't just about looking after your teeth. It's about preserving your ability to enjoy life, communicate, eat well, and express yourself with confidence. With proper care, your natural teeth can last a lifetime as its designed to stay lifelong.

When to Visit a Dentist:

It's recommended to visit a dentist regularly and whenever you notice any issues with your oral cavity.

Here' s a quick guide:

- Routine Check-ups: Every six months for cleanings and check-ups.

- Children: First dental visit by age one or when the first tooth erupts.

Symptoms to Watch For:

- Toothache or sensitivity

- Swollen, bleeding, or red gums

- Persistent bad breath or bad taste

- Loose teeth or changes in bite

- Sores, lumps, or white/red patches in the mouth

Dental Visits at Every Stage of Life:

Whether you're caring for a child's first tooth, a teenager's developing smile, or your own teeth as you grow older, dental visits play an essential role in maintaining oral health and overall well-being. Here's when you should see your dentist—and why it matters at every age.

Infants and Toddlers: The First Tooth

• First Visit: Children should see a dentist by the time their first tooth appears or by age one.

• Purpose: Early visits ensure healthy development, teach parents about oral hygiene for infants, and allow the dentist to monitor for any issues with alignment, teething, or decay.

Children and Adolescents: Building Healthy Habits

• Regular Visits (Every Six Months): Preventive care, including cleanings and fluoride treatments, helps maintain healthy teeth as children grow.

- Purpose: Dentists monitor for cavities, gum health, and alignment issues. Early detection of issues like crowded or misaligned teeth allows for timely intervention, often with orthodontics.

- Education: Teaching kids the importance of brushing, flossing, and making healthy food choices lays the foundation for lifelong habits.

Teenagers: Orthodontics and Wisdom Teeth

- Routine Check-ups: Continue every six months, with a focus on maintaining good hygiene and addressing any specific issues related to puberty and hormonal changes.

- Orthodontic Evaluations: Often necessary during adolescence to correct alignment or bite issues.

- Wisdom Teeth Assessment: Dentists will monitor the development of wisdom teeth, which typically emerge in the late teens or early twenties, to determine if extraction is needed to prevent overcrowding or impaction.

Adults: Ongoing Maintenance and Preventive Care

- Biannual Visits for Cleanings and Check-ups: Essential for detecting cavities, gum disease, and early signs of oral cancer.

- Purpose: Dentists can identify potential problems before they escalate, often saving time, expense, and discomfort.

- Periodontal Health: With age, gum health becomes even more important. Gum disease is a leading cause of tooth loss in adults and can affect overall health, linking to conditions like heart disease and diabetes.

• Oral Cancer Screenings: Adults should have regular screenings for early detection of oral cancer, which is most treatable when identified early.

Pregnant Women: Specialized Dental Care

• Regular Visits: Essential during pregnancy, as hormonal changes can increase the risk of gum disease and pregnancy gingivitis.

• Purpose: Maintaining good oral health during pregnancy is linked to better outcomes for both mother and baby, reducing the risk of preterm birth and other complications.

Older Adults: Preserving Natural Teeth and Oral Health

• Regular Visits: Older adults should continue biannual check-ups and cleanings.

• Focus on Retaining Natural Teeth: With proper care, natural teeth can often be maintained well into old age.

• Dental Care for Dentures and Implants: Regular visits are essential, even for those with dentures or implants, to ensure they fit comfortably, prevent sores, and monitor for any other oral health issues.

• Dry Mouth and Medications: Many older adults experience dry mouth due to medications, which increases the risk of decay and gum disease. Dentists can provide guidance and solutions to manage this condition.

Visiting the dentist regularly at every stage of life can make profound difference, not just for your teeth but for your quality of life. A healthy mouth supports a healthy body, and routine dental visits allow us to catch problems early, support overall wellness, and help each generation keep their natural smile for as long as possible.

As my patient's story reminds us, dental care is an investment in our future. Whether you're just starting out with a child's first tooth or maintaining your own oral health well into your golden years, regular dental care is the foundation of a lifetime of smiles.

Chapter 9

Shedding and Eruption Timeline

It is important to know clear shedding and eruption timeline of baby teeth and permanent teeth, organized to help parents understand when each type of tooth generally falls out and when adult teeth emerge. In some cases, the milk teeth or temporary teeth also called deciduous teeth fails to fall on time and leads crowding that permanent tooth tends to erupt in wrong position. Knowledge on eruption and shedding timeline helps parents to arrange dental visit in case the child need an extraction, so space allow to erupt permanent teeth in right position.

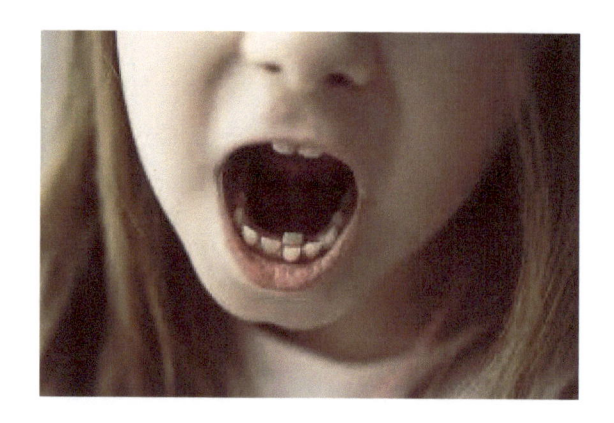

Baby (Primary) Teeth Shedding Timeline:

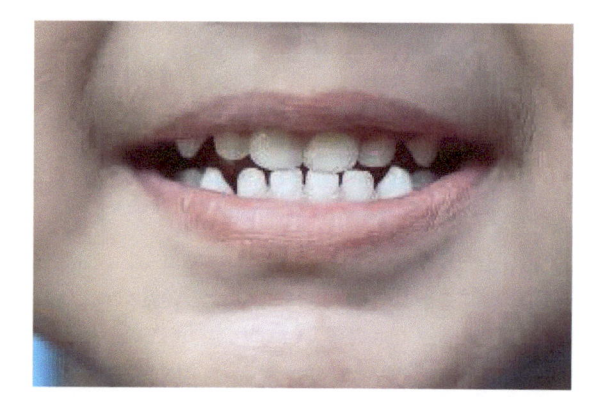

- 6 to 7 years: Central incisors (front teeth) – both upper and lower

- 7 to 8 years: Lateral incisors (next to central incisors) – both upper and lower

- 9 to 11 years: First molars (back teeth used for grinding food)

- 10 to 12 years: Canines (pointed teeth next to lateral incisors)
- 10 to 12 years: Second molars (the last of the baby teeth to be shed)

Permanent (Adult) Teeth Eruption Timeline:

- 6 to 7 years: First molars (back teeth that don't replace any baby teeth but come in as new teeth)
- 6 to 7 years: Lower central incisors (front bottom teeth)
- 7 to 8 years: Upper central incisors (front top teeth)
- 7 to 8 years: Lower lateral incisors (next to central incisors on the bottom)
- 8 to 9 years: Upper lateral incisors (next to central incisors on the top)
- 9 to 10 years: Lower canines (pointed teeth next to lateral incisors)
- 10 to 11 years: Upper first premolars (replacing baby molars)

- 10 to 12 years: Lower first premolars (replacing baby molars)
- 11 to 12 years: Upper second premolars (replacing baby molars)
- 11 to 12 years: Lower second premolars (replacing baby molars)
- 11 to 12 years: Upper canines (pointed teeth next to lateral incisors)
- 12 to 13 years: Second molars (back teeth)
- 17 to 21 years: Third molars (wisdom teeth, if they erupt)

Tooth Eruption Chart

Primary Teeth

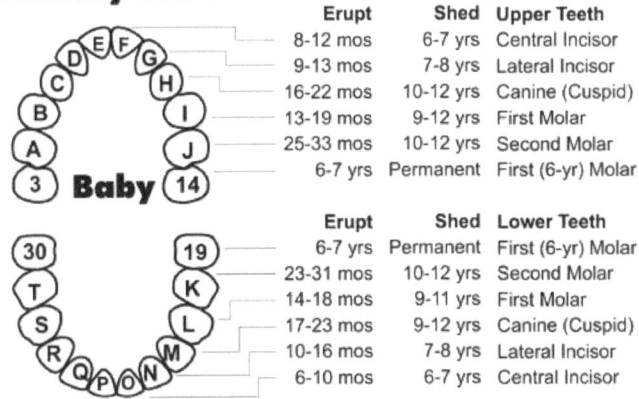

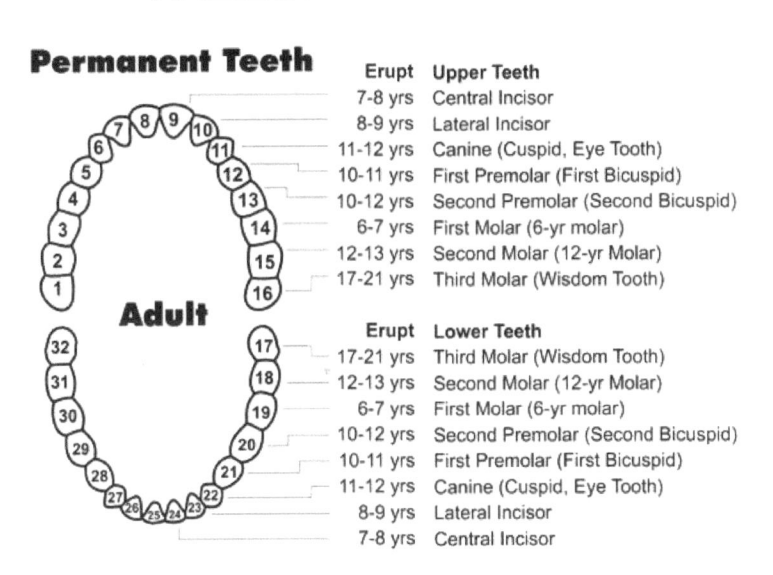

	Erupt	Shed	Upper Teeth
	8-12 mos	6-7 yrs	Central Incisor
	9-13 mos	7-8 yrs	Lateral Incisor
	16-22 mos	10-12 yrs	Canine (Cuspid)
	13-19 mos	9-12 yrs	First Molar
	25-33 mos	10-12 yrs	Second Molar
	6-7 yrs	Permanent	First (6-yr) Molar

	Erupt	Shed	Lower Teeth
	6-7 yrs	Permanent	First (6-yr) Molar
	23-31 mos	10-12 yrs	Second Molar
	14-18 mos	9-11 yrs	First Molar
	17-23 mos	9-12 yrs	Canine (Cuspid)
	10-16 mos	7-8 yrs	Lateral Incisor
	6-10 mos	6-7 yrs	Central Incisor

Permanent Teeth

Erupt	Upper Teeth
7-8 yrs	Central Incisor
8-9 yrs	Lateral Incisor
11-12 yrs	Canine (Cuspid, Eye Tooth)
10-11 yrs	First Premolar (First Bicuspid)
10-12 yrs	Second Premolar (Second Bicuspid)
6-7 yrs	First Molar (6-yr molar)
12-13 yrs	Second Molar (12-yr Molar)
17-21 yrs	Third Molar (Wisdom Tooth)

Erupt	Lower Teeth
17-21 yrs	Third Molar (Wisdom Tooth)
12-13 yrs	Second Molar (12-yr Molar)
6-7 yrs	First Molar (6-yr molar)
10-12 yrs	Second Premolar (Second Bicuspid)
10-11 yrs	First Premolar (First Bicuspid)
11-12 yrs	Canine (Cuspid, Eye Tooth)
8-9 yrs	Lateral Incisor
7-8 yrs	Central Incisor

Additional Tips for Parents:

- Baby teeth usually start shedding around age 6 and finish by age 12, when most of the permanent teeth have erupted.

- Regular dental check-ups allow monitoring of each stage to ensure teeth are shedding and erupting on time and in the correct alignment.

- Encouraging good oral hygiene habits with both baby and permanent teeth supports the health of adult teeth as they come in.

This timeline can give parents a helpful guide to know what to expect and ensure their child's dental development is on track.

The Ugly Duckling Stage:

The "ugly duckling stage" or "Mixed Dentition" is a normal developmental phase typically seen in children between the ages of 7 and 12. During this period, the following characteristics are common:

1. **Gapped Front Teeth (Diastema):**

- A noticeable gap often appears between the upper central incisors (front teeth) due to the growth of the jaw and positioning of adjacent teeth.

2. **Angled Canines:**

- The permanent canines begin to erupt and put pressure on the roots of the central and lateral incisors, causing them to angle outward.

3. **Temporary Misalignment:**

- The overall appearance may look crowded, gapped, or uneven, giving the "ugly duckling" look. This is typically a natural, self-correcting phase.

4. **Correction:**

- As the canines and other teeth fully erupt, they tend to push the front teeth back into proper alignment, closing gaps and straightening any temporary misalignments.

5. OPG (Orthopantomogram) of Mixed Dentition or Ugly duckling stage look like:

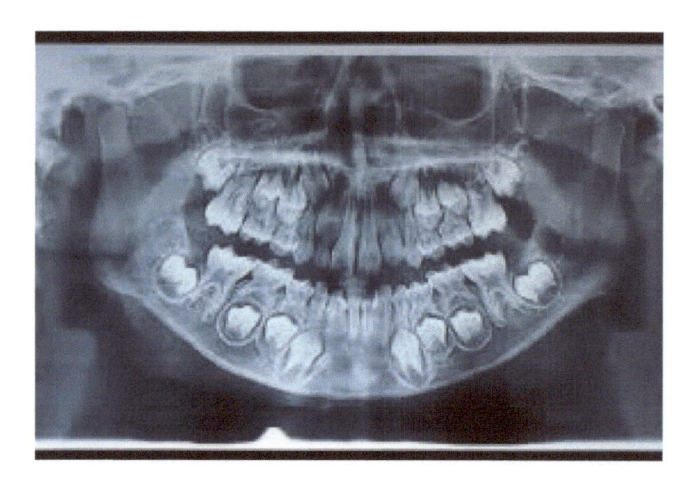

The "ugly duckling stage" is a normal part of dental development. This stage often resolves naturally, but it's still helpful to have regular dental check-ups during this time to monitor for proper alignment and intervene only if necessary.

Chapter 10

Oral Cavity – Know Me Well

What is the Oral Cavity?

The oral cavity, often called the mouth, is the entryway to the digestive and respiratory systems. It plays a vital role in eating, speaking, breathing, and expressing emotions.

The oral cavity isn't just about teeth; it includes various structures that work together to support essential functions. Let's break it down into parts and functions to help understand each component and why they are important for overall health.

Structures of the Oral Cavity

The oral cavity can be divided into two main parts:

- Vestibule: The area between the lips/cheeks and the teeth.

- Oral Cavity Proper: The area inside the teeth and gums, extending to the throat.

Here's a look at each major structure:

a. Lips and Cheeks
   - Lips are the soft outer part of the mouth that help with speech and keep food and saliva inside while eating.
   - Cheeks form the sides of the mouth, made up of muscles that help in chewing, smiling, and speaking.

Together, the lips and cheeks play a role in forming facial expressions, keeping the mouth moist, and controlling food and air intake.

b. Teeth
   - Teeth are hard, calcified structures embedded in the gums. Humans have two sets:
   - Primary (baby) teeth: 20 teeth that come in during childhood.
   - Permanent teeth: 32 teeth that replace the baby teeth and should ideally last a lifetime.

Teeth are used to chew (break down) food into small pieces for digestion and play an important role in speaking clearly. They also help shape the face.

Types of teeth:

- Incisors: The flat, sharp teeth in the front that cut food.
- Canines: Pointed teeth next to the incisors for tearing food.
- Premolars and Molars: Located in the back, these have flat surfaces for grinding and chewing.

c. Gums (Gingiva)
  - Gums are soft, Coral pink tissues that surround and support the teeth. They protect the roots and bones that hold the teeth in place. Healthy gums are firm and Coral pink, and they play a crucial role in protecting teeth from bacteria.

d. Tongue
  - The tongue is a muscular organ covered in taste buds that detect flavors (sweet, salty, sour, bitter).
  - It helps in speaking, chewing, and swallowing food by moving it around in the mouth.
  - The tongue also helps clean the teeth and mixes saliva with food for easier digestion.

e. Salivary Glands
  - Salivary glands produce saliva, which helps moisten food, making it easier to chew and swallow.
  - Saliva contains enzymes that start breaking down food, especially starches, and helps keep the mouth clean by washing away food particles and bacteria.

There are three major pairs of salivary glands:

- Parotid glands (near the ear)
- Submandibular glands (under the jaw)
- Sublingual glands (under the tongue)

f. Hard and Soft Palate

- The hard palate is the bony front part of the roof of the mouth. It provides a hard surface for the tongue to press against when chewing and speaking.
- The soft palate is the soft, flexible back part of the roof of the mouth. It helps close off the nasal passages during swallowing so food doesn't go up into the nose.

The uvula (the small piece of tissue that hangs down at the back of the soft palate) plays a role in speech and swallowing.

g. Throat (Pharynx)

- The pharynx connects the mouth to the oesophagus and the nasal passages, allowing food to pass into the digestive tract and air to pass into the respiratory tract. It plays a role in both breathing and swallowing.

Functions of the Oral Cavity

The oral cavity is involved in several essential functions:

- Digestion: The mouth is where digestion begins. Teeth break down food, the tongue and cheeks help move it around, and saliva starts the chemical breakdown.

- Speech: Teeth, tongue, and palate work together to create sounds and articulate words.

- Breathing: The mouth serves as a secondary passage for air intake, especially when the nose is blocked.

- Protection: Saliva helps to wash away bacteria and food particles, protecting the mouth from infections.

- Taste: Taste buds on the tongue detect flavors, enhancing the enjoyment of food and helping to identify spoiled or harmful substances.

Understanding the structures and functions of the oral cavity highlights why it's essential to care for this part of the body. Oral health not only affects your smile but also your ability to eat, speak, and stay healthy.

Chapter 11

Dental Team – A Family

The dental team is made up of several professionals who work together to ensure that patients receive comprehensive and high-quality dental care. Each member plays a specific role, and together, they cover everything from preventive care and diagnosis to treatment and patient education.

Here's an overview of who is typically included in a dental team and their roles:

1. Dentist (General or Specialist)

- Role: The dentist is the primary dental care provider and often leads the dental team. They diagnose and treat oral diseases, perform procedures (like fillings, crowns, root canals, and extractions), and oversee the overall dental health of patients.

- Training: Dentists complete a Doctor of Dental Surgery (DDS) or Doctor of Dental Medicine (DMD) degree or Bachelor's in dental surgery (BDS), which usually requires 5 years of dental school after completing undergraduate studies.
- Specialists: Dentists may further specialize in areas such as:
  - Orthodontics (alignment of teeth and jaws)
  - Periodontics (gums and supporting structures)
  - Endodontics (root canal therapy)
  - Oral Surgery (surgical procedures like extractions and implants)
  - Prosthodontics (dental prosthetics, such as crowns, bridges, and dentures)
  - Pediatric Dentistry (dental care for children)
  - Oral and Maxillofacial Radiology (diagnostic imaging of facial structures)

2. Dental Hygienist

- Role: Dental hygienists focus on preventive oral care. They clean patients' teeth, take X-rays, apply sealants and fluoride, and provide education on proper oral hygiene.
- Training: Most dental hygienists complete an associate or bachelor's degree in dental hygiene and are licensed

to practice.

- Scope: Hygienists work closely with patients to prevent gum disease and tooth decay by cleaning the teeth and providing individualized oral hygiene instructions.

3. Dental Assistant

- Role: Dental assistants support both the dentist and the hygienist in clinical tasks. They prepare patients for treatments, assist during procedures, sterilize instruments, take X-rays, and manage the patient's dental records.
- Training: Training varies by region and may range from on-the-job training to formal certification programs.
- Patient Interaction: Dental assistants often help make patients comfortable, explain procedures, and provide aftercare instructions.

4. Dental Laboratory Technician

- Role: Dental technicians work behind the scenes to create dental appliances based on a dentist's specifications. This includes crowns, bridges, dentures, orthodontic appliances, and custom mouth-guards.
- Training: They typically complete specialized training in dental laboratory technology, which may be through an accredited program or an apprenticeship.
- Artistic and Technical Skills: Dental lab technicians use materials like ceramics, metal, and acrylics to create realistic and functional restorations.

5. Receptionist or Administrative Staff

- Role: The receptionist or administrative staff handles the non-clinical aspects of a dental office. They schedule appointments, manage patient records, handle billing and insurance claims, and ensure smooth communication within the office.
- Patient Interaction: Receptionists are often the first point of contact, welcoming patients, answering questions, and facilitating the administrative side of their care.

6. Dental Therapist (in some countries)

- Role: A dental therapist is trained to provide a limited range of dental services, including basic restorative care (like fillings), preventive care, and extractions of baby teeth. They work under the supervision of a dentist and often provide care to underserved populations.
- Training: Training requirements **vary** but generally include specialized programs focused on essential procedures.
- Scope: Dental therapists help increase access to care, particularly perform a variety of routine and restorative dental procedures and provide oral health education.

7. Oral Health Educator

- Role: While not always part of every dental team, some practices employ oral health educators to focus on patient education, prevention programs, and public awareness about oral health.
- Training: They may be trained dental hygienists, therapists or assistants who specialize in public health education.

- Community Outreach: Oral health educators often work with schools, public health departments, and community programs to promote dental health.

8. **Periodontal Therapist (sometimes integrated into a hygienist's role)**
    - Role: A periodontal therapist is specially trained to provide non-surgical periodontal (gum) treatments, including scaling, root planing, and maintenance for patients with gum disease.
    - Training: Often, this is an additional role or training undertaken by dental hygienists to focus specifically on the health of the gums and supporting structures of the teeth.
    - Scope: Their work is crucial for preventing and managing periodontal disease, which can have significant impacts on overall health.

Summary of the Dental Teams Goals:

The dental team works together to provide comprehensive oral care. Their goals include:

1. Preventive Care: Helping patients avoid oral health problems through education, routine cleanings, and assessments.

2. Diagnostic Care: Identifying and diagnosing oral health issues early to prevent complications.

3. Restorative Care: Restoring damaged teeth and tissues to improve function and appearance.

4. Surgical Care: Performing necessary surgeries, from extractions to implants, to address complex dental issues.

5. Patient Education: Ensuring patients understand their treatment plans, oral hygiene practices, and how to maintain oral health.

Every member of the dental team has a specific role, also every member will be trained for CPR (Cardiac pulmonary resuscitation) and medical emergencies, and they collaborate to ensure each patient receives high-quality care in a supportive and comfortable environment.

Chapter 12

Do Medical Histories Matter in Dental Care?

"Patients often wonder why we ask for detailed medical histories, even for a routine hygiene visit or dental check-up. However, knowing your medical background is essential for safe and effective care.

Dental procedures, even minor ones, involve physical stressors like air and water, which can affect individuals differently based on their health conditions. Patients often find it unimportant to discuss medical histories which leads to stressing them questioning on allergies or any current treatment if they are upto as they declare all nil on clinipad or medical history form.

For instance, patients with a history of anxiety, high blood pressure, epilepsy, or allergies may be at a higher risk of complications during treatment. By understanding your medical history and any medications you're on, we can proactively adjust our approach, prevent potential emergencies, and provide any necessary post-care. This comprehensive information allows us to ensure your visit is as comfortable and safe as possible."

Gathering a patient's full medical history is crucial in dental care for safe and effective treatment. Certain conditions and medications can directly impact dental procedures, influencing treatment choices and emergency preparedness.

Why Medical Histories Matter:

1. Medication Interactions: Some medications, like blood thinners, can increase bleeding risk during dental procedures.

2. Medical Conditions: Conditions such as epilepsy, high blood pressure, diabetes, or anxiety disorders can increase the likelihood of dental chair emergencies.

3. Allergies: Knowledge of allergies (e.g., to latex or anesthesia) helps prevent severe allergic reactions.

4. Anxiety and Stress Sensitivity: Patients prone to anxiety attacks may need additional support or treatment modifications to prevent undue stress.

Conditions That Could Lead to Dental Emergencies:

- Cardiovascular Issues: Patients with high blood pressure or heart conditions may experience stress-induced complications.

- Diabetes: Blood sugar levels can fluctuate, impacting healing and risk for infection.

- Respiratory Conditions: Conditions like asthma may worsen under stress or due to dental sprays and tools.

Certain medical conditions can impact the safe use and effectiveness of local anesthesia in dental procedures. Here are some key conditions to be aware of:

1. Heart Conditions: Patients with cardiovascular diseases, especially those on blood pressure or anti-arrhythmic medications, may be at risk since some anesthetics contain epinephrine, which can raise blood pressure and heart rate.

2. Respiratory Disorders: Conditions like asthma or chronic obstructive pulmonary disease (COPD) may worsen under sedation or local anesthesia.

3. Liver or kidney disease: These organs are essential in processing anesthetic drugs. Impaired liver or kidney

function can lead to slower drug clearance and prolonged effects of anesthesia.

4. Allergies: Allergies to local anesthetic components, though rare, can cause severe reactions, so allergy history is crucial.

5. Diabetes: Diabetics can experience fluctuations in blood sugar levels, especially with the stress of procedures, and anesthesia might affect glucose metabolism.

6. Thyroid Disorders: Hyperthyroidism can interact with epinephrine-containing anesthetics, increasing the risk of adverse cardiovascular reactions.

7. Pregnancy: Pregnant patients should generally avoid certain anesthetics due to potential risks to the fetus. Also, patients those who have done IVF (in vitro fertilization) and are waiting to conceive should always inform dental professionals. It's recommended not to do any dental treatment that cause physical stress or mental stress until the confirmation of pregnancy.

Informing the dental team about these conditions ensures they can adjust the type and dosage of anesthesia to ensure safety and comfort.

Most Commonly asked questions in Medical History Form:

Health conditions:

- Breathing problems, such as asthma or bronchitis
- Heart problems, such as angina, blood pressure, or stroke
- Diabetes or family history of diabetes
- Bone or joint disease
- Liver or kidney disease
- Any other serious illnesses or infectious diseases

Medications

- What medications are you taking, including name, dose, and frequency
- Have you ever had a bad reaction to a general or local anesthetic?

Risk factors

- Do you smoke tobacco products, vape, or chew tobacco?
- Do you have a family history of heart disease?
- Do you have a history of fainting attacks, epilepsy, or blackouts?

Knowing a patient's medical history allows the dental team to proactively manage risks, ensure the use of appropriate materials, and provide post-care instructions tailored to individual health needs.

Chapter 13

I am Old, and so is My Tooth!

An elderly patient recently shared a touching dream with me. She had seen her teeth talking to each other, mourning their end. In her dream, the canine said to the molar, "I help shape the lips and cut food, but still, I feel overlooked." As she prepared to say goodbye to her last teeth and transition to complete dentures, she expressed a mix of humor and sadness.

It was clear that, despite her jokes, losing her teeth felt like losing a part of herself. When she mentioned she wouldn't need future visits, I gently reminded her that dental exams still matter, even without natural teeth, for monitoring her full oral health. Our role goes beyond just teeth—we're here to care for the entire mouth, watching for any early signs of issues, like precancerous lesions or other conditions.

Her story stayed with me. It reminded me of the deep emotional ties we have with our teeth and the importance of providing compassionate care, even when patients feel they no longer "need" us. I encouraged her to visit, not just for health, but for the connection and reassurance that we're here for her teeth or no teeth.

As we age, regular dental check-ups are essential for monitoring early signs of precancerous oral lesions or conditions. Here are key signs and symptoms to be aware of, particularly for those over 50:

1. White or Red Patches: Persistent white (leukoplakia) or red (erythroplakia) patches on the gums, tongue, or lining of the mouth could be early indicators of abnormal cell growth.

Pictures below shows white or red patches which can be Leukoplakia or erythroplakia:

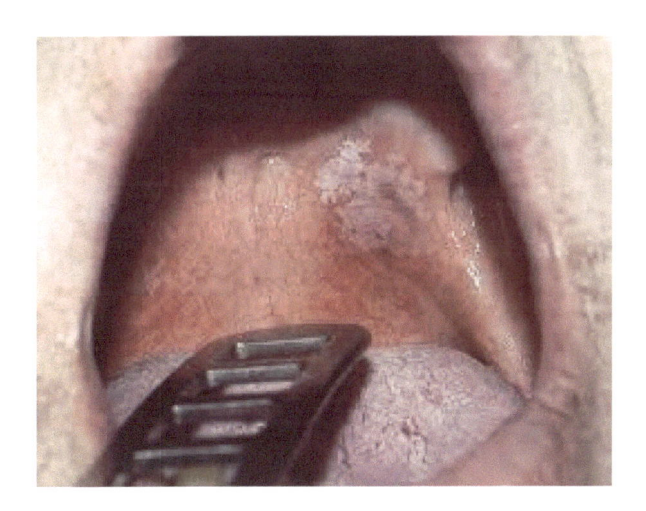

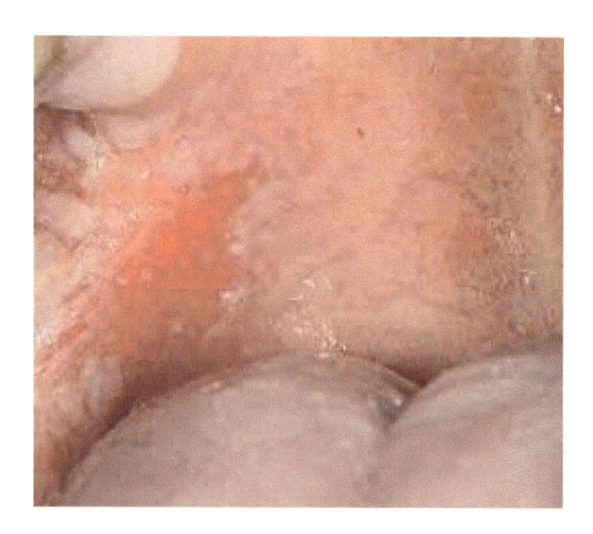

2. Non-Healing Sores: Mouth sores that don't heal within two weeks or that bleed easily should be checked by a dental professional.

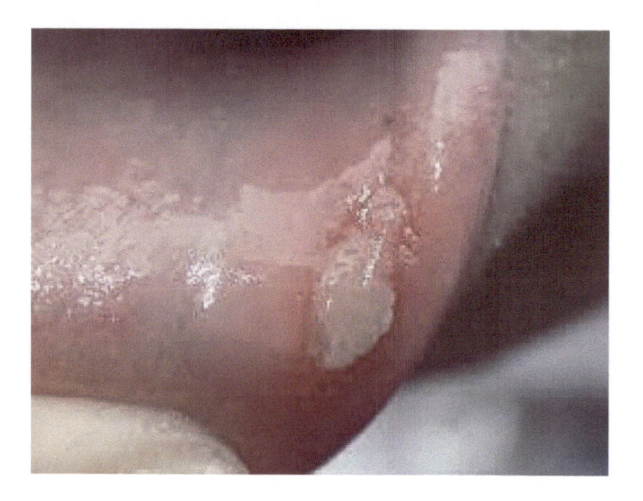

3. Lumps or Thickened Areas: Any lumps, thickened spots, or rough areas in the mouth, throat, or cheeks could indicate underlying conditions.

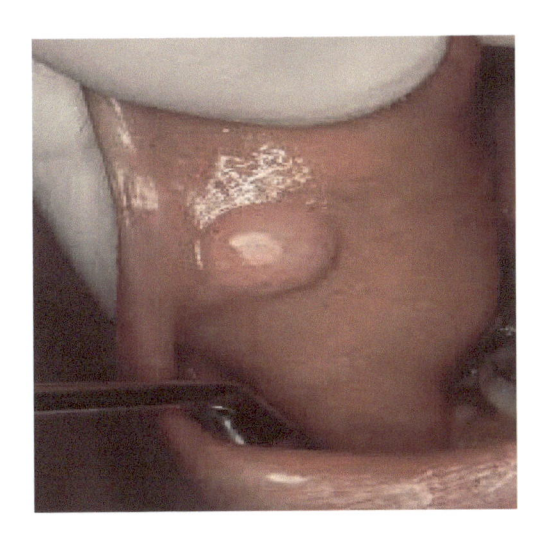

4. Difficulty Swallowing or Chewing: Trouble moving the jaw or tongue or persistent sore throat can be signs of potential issues.

5. Numbness or Pain: Persistent numbness, pain, or tenderness in the mouth or face is also a red flag.

These symptoms don't always indicate cancer, but they're worth discussing with a dentist to catch any issues early. Regular exams allow professionals to monitor changes and detect potential risks promptly.

Chapter 14

I Am Your Tooth – What's My Role?

1. Incisors:

These front teeth (eight total—four on top and four on the bottom) have sharp, thin edges for cutting food. They are essential to the smile and play a key role in speech, particularly in sounds like "F" and "V." Incisors also support the lips and help maintain proper jaw alignment.

2. Canines:

Located next to the incisors, these pointed teeth (four total) tear food and help shape the lips, enhancing the arc of the smile.

3. Premolars (Bicuspids):

Behind the canines, premolars (eight total) have flat surfaces for crushing, tearing, and grinding food. They maintain facial height, support cheek muscles, and are visible in the smile, although less prominently than incisors and canines.

4. Molars:

At the back, molars (twelve total, including wisdom teeth) have large, flat surfaces for grinding food to aid digestion. Molars are crucial for jaw balance, as they distribute chewing force evenly, preventing excessive pressure on other teeth. They also play a key role in occlusion, ensuring proper jaw alignment when the mouth closes.

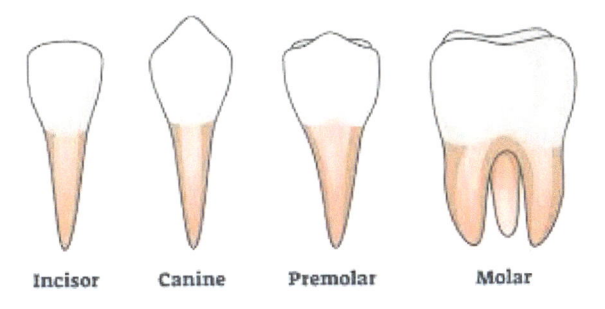

Incisor　　Canine　　Premolar　　Molar

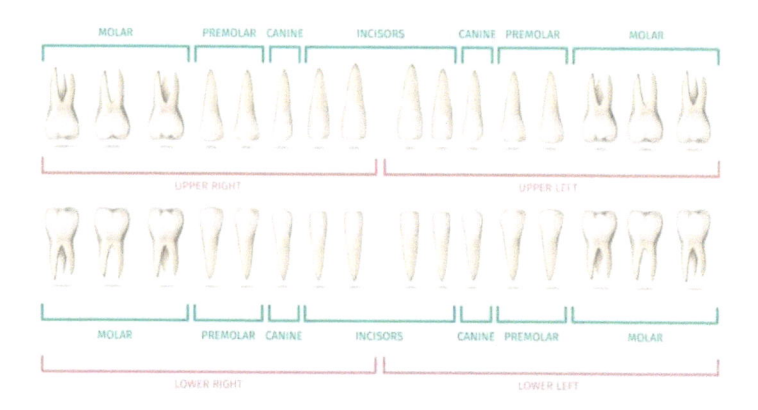

Together, these teeth enable efficient chewing, clear speech, and support proper jaw alignment.

Miscellaneous Oral cavity Atlas

Structure of oral cavity:

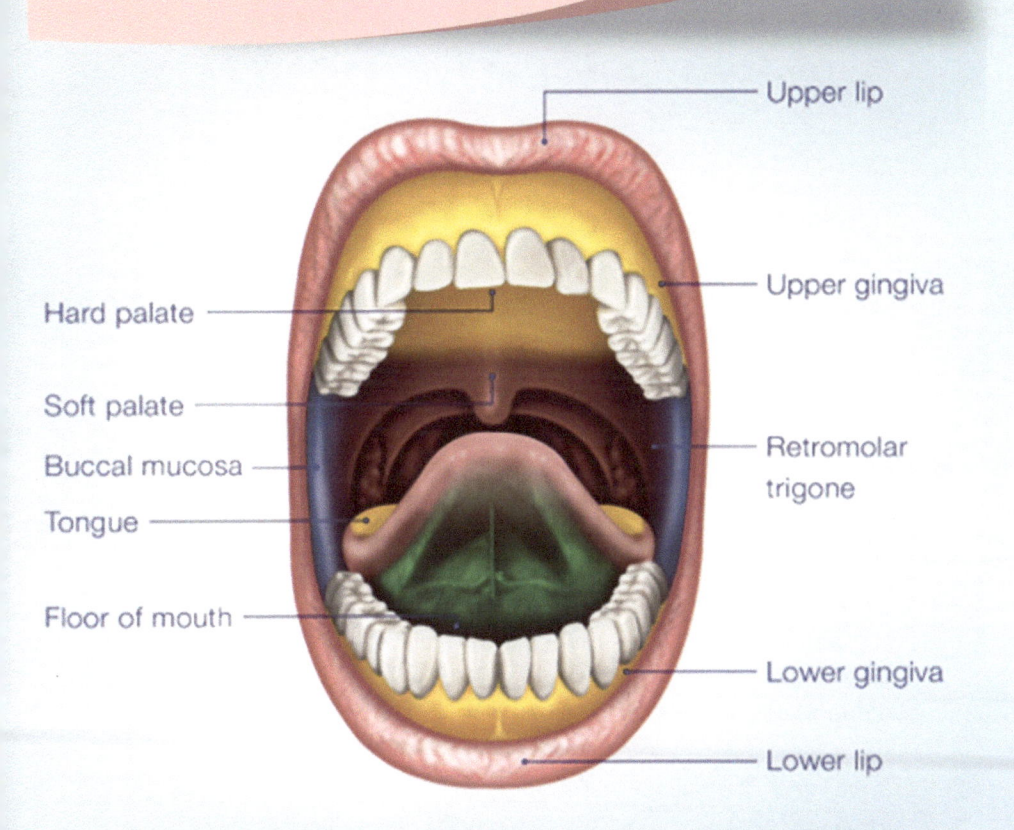

- Upper lip
- Upper gingiva
- Hard palate
- Soft palate
- Buccal mucosa
- Tongue
- Retromolar trigone
- Floor of mouth
- Lower gingiva
- Lower lip

Tooth Anatomy

Tooth Anatomy

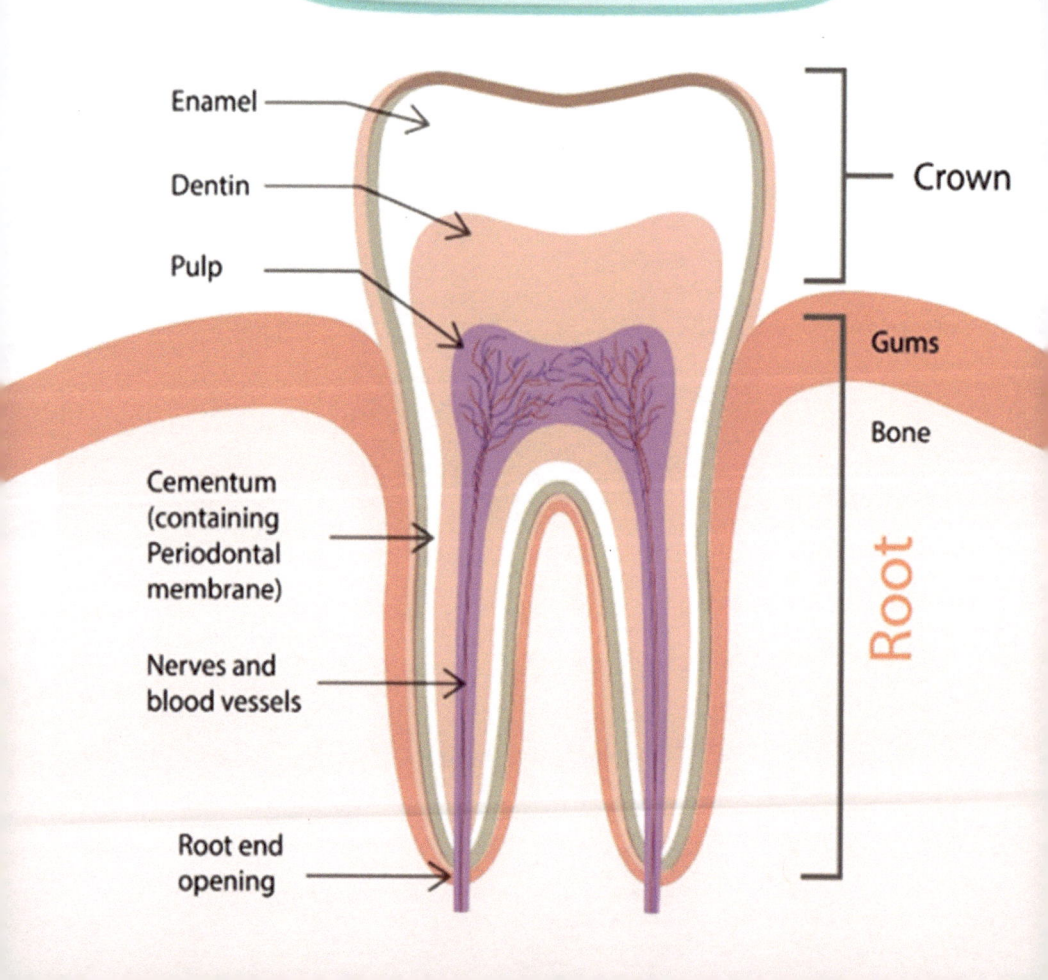

- Enamel
- Dentin
- Pulp
- Cementum (containing Periodontal membrane)
- Nerves and blood vessels
- Root end opening

- Crown
- Gums
- Bone
- Root

Dental Plaque

DENTAL BIOFILM (PLAQUE)

HEALTHY TOOTH TOOTH WITH DENTAL BIOFILM (PLAQUE)

Dental plaque is a sticky, colourless film of bacteria that forms on teeth. Over time, if not removed through proper oral hygiene, it can harden into tartar and lead to dental issues such as cavities and gum disease.

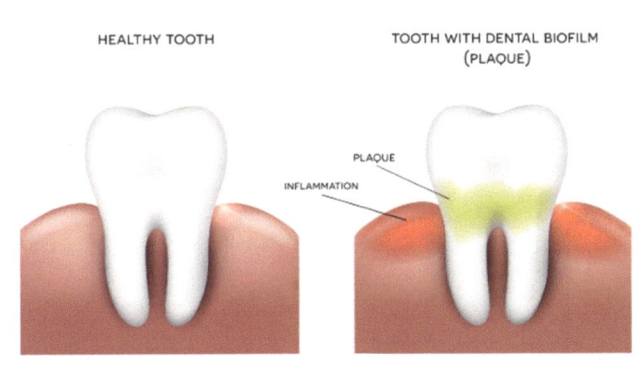

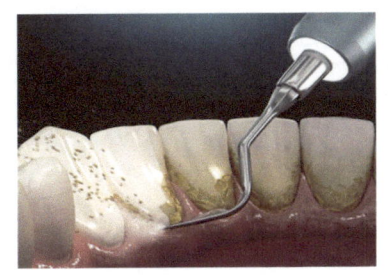

Understanding the stages of dental plaque formation is crucial for maintaining oral health. Plaque development progresses through several phases:

1. **Pellicle Formation:** A protein film forms on the tooth surface within minutes after cleaning.
2. **Initial Bacterial Colonization:** Early colonizers, primarily gram-positive cocci, adhere to the pellicle.
3. **Secondary Colonization and Plaque Maturation:** Diverse bacterial species coaggregate, leading to a complex biofilm.

The stages of periodontal disease

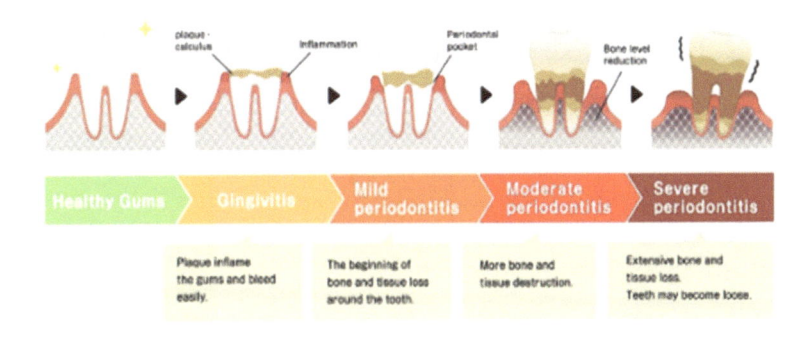

Healthy Gums	Gingivitis	Mild periodontitis	Moderate periodontitis	Severe periodontitis
	Plaque inflame the gums and bleed easily.	The beginning of bone and tissue loss around the tooth.	More bone and tissue destruction.	Extensive bone and tissue loss. Teeth may become loose.

Enamel Demineralization

Enamel demineralization is the initial stage of tooth decay, characterized by the loss of essential minerals like calcium and phosphate from the tooth's enamel surface. This process often manifests as white spots on the teeth, indicating areas where the enamel has begun to weaken.

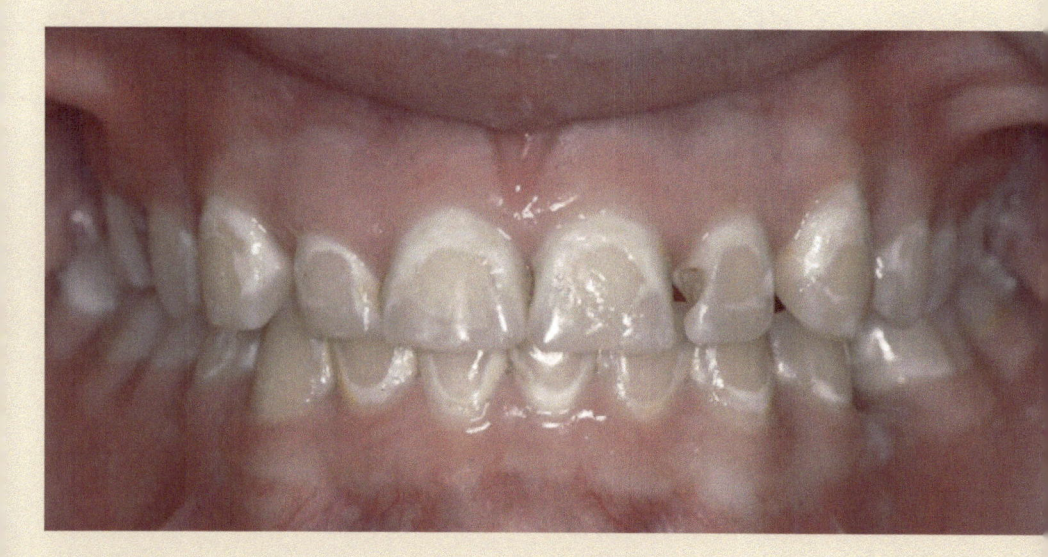

To prevent and manage enamel demineralization:

- **Maintain Proper Oral Hygiene**: Brush twice daily with fluoride toothpaste and floss regularly to remove plaque.
- **Limit Sugary and Acidic Foods**: Reduce consumption of foods and beverages high in sugar and acid, as they contribute to enamel erosion.
- **Regular Dental Check-ups:** Visit your dentist routinely for professional cleanings and early detection of potential issues.

Addressing enamel demineralization promptly can prevent further tooth decay and maintain overall oral health.

Stages of tooth decay:

Understanding the stages of tooth decay is crucial for effective prevention and treatment. Here's an overview of each stage:

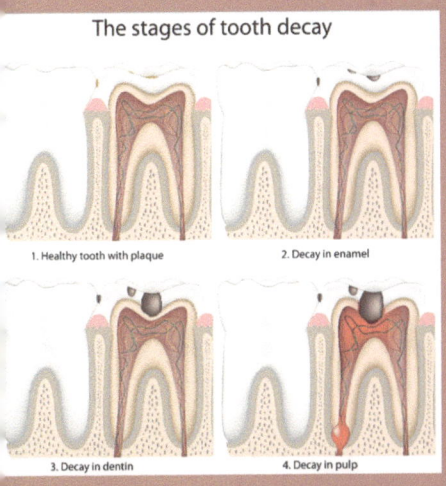

1. White Spots (Initial Demineralization):
- Description: Early signs include chalky white areas on the tooth surface, indicating mineral loss due to acid-producing bacteria.
- Reversibility: At this stage, decay can be halted or reversed with proper oral hygiene and fluoride treatments.

2. Enamel Decay:
- Description: The enamel begins to break down, leading to the formation of small cavities.
- Treatment: Professional intervention is required to fill cavities and prevent further decay.

3. Dentin Decay:
- Description: Decay progresses beyond the enamel into the dentin, the layer beneath. This can cause increased sensitivity.
- Treatment: More extensive fillings or restorative procedures may be necessary.

4. Pulp Damage:
- Description: The decay reaches the tooth's pulp, containing nerves and blood vessels, leading to pain and potential infection.
- Treatment: Root canal therapy is often required to remove infected tissue and save the tooth.

5. Abscess Formation:
- Description: An abscess, a pocket of pus, forms at the tooth's root due to bacterial infection, causing severe pain and swelling.
- Treatment: Immediate dental treatment is essential, which may include drainage, antibiotics, or tooth extraction.

Dental Abscess:

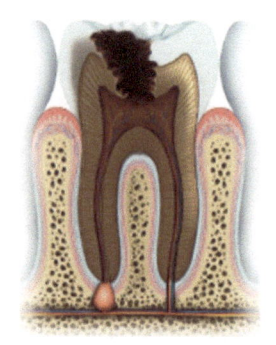

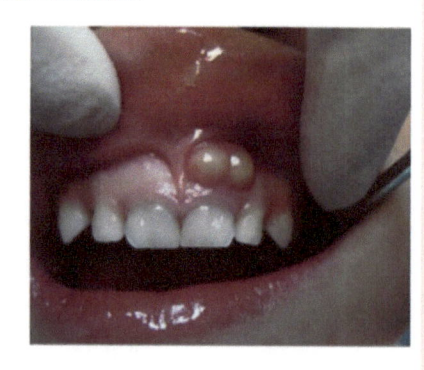

A dental abscess is a collection of pus that forms in or around a tooth due to a bacterial infection. This infection can occur in different areas near the tooth for various reasons:

- **Periapical Abscess:** Occurs at the tip of the tooth's root, often resulting from untreated dental cavities, injury, or prior dental work.
- **Periodontal Abscess:** Affects the gums and supporting bone structure, typically due to gum disease.

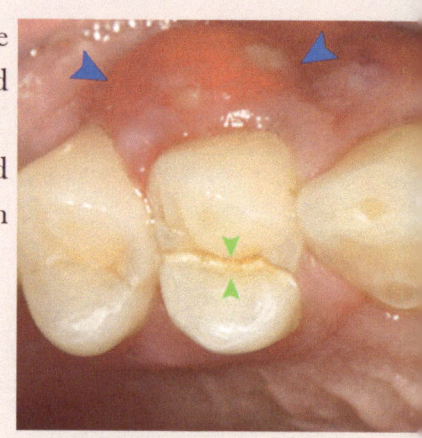

Common Symptoms:

- Severe, throbbing toothache that can radiate to the jawbone, neck, or ear.
- Sensitivity to hot and cold temperatures.
- Swelling in the face, cheek, or neck.
- Tender, swollen lymph nodes under the jaw or in the neck.
- Foul odor in the mouth.
- Difficulty opening the mouth or swallowing.

It's crucial to seek prompt dental care if you suspect an abscess, as the infection can spread to other parts of the body, leading to serious complications.

Non-Carious tooth surface loss:

Understanding the differences between dental attrition, abrasion, and erosion is essential for maintaining oral health. Each condition affects the teeth in distinct ways:

1. Attrition: This refers to the gradual wearing down of tooth surfaces due to tooth-to-tooth contact, commonly resulting from habits like grinding or clenching.

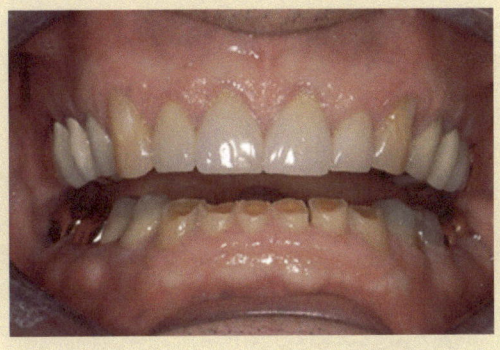

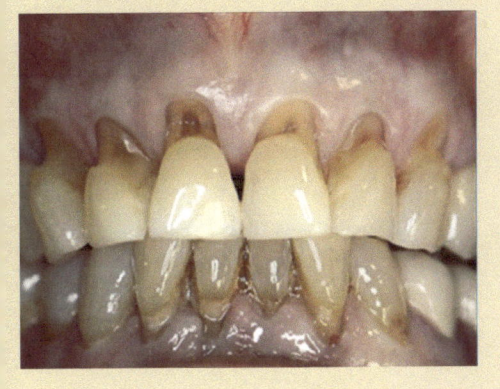

2. Abrasion: This involves the loss of tooth structure caused by external mechanical forces, such as aggressive tooth brushing or using abrasive dental products.

3. Erosion: This is the chemical dissolution of tooth enamel due to exposure to acids from dietary sources or gastric reflux, leading to a smooth, scooped-out appearance on the tooth surface.

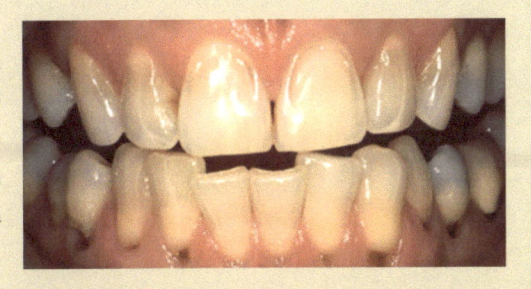

Rampant Caries and Nursing bottle caries:

Rampant caries and nursing bottle caries (also known as early childhood caries) are two terms often used in dentistry to describe specific patterns of severe tooth decay. While they share some similarities, there are distinct differences:

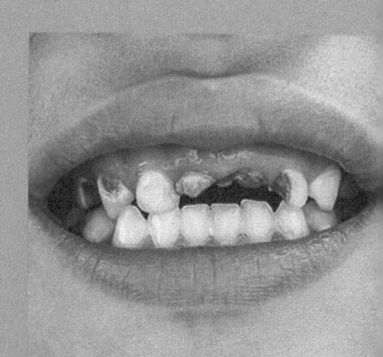

Rampant Caries:

- **Definition:** A severe and widespread form of tooth decay that affects multiple teeth rapidly, regardless of the patient's age.
- **Causes:**
- Poor oral hygiene.
- High sugar or carbohydrate consumption.
- Xerostomia (dry mouth), often caused by medications, radiation therapy, or systemic conditions.
- Substance abuse, such as methamphetamine use (commonly called "meth mouth").
- **Affected Population:** Can occur in any age group, including children, teenagers, and adults.
- **Tooth Involvement:**

Affects multiple teeth, often including anterior and posterior teeth.

May progress quickly, involving both enamel and dentin.

- **Risk Factors:**

Poor dietary habits.

Inadequate fluoride exposure.

Systemic diseases or treatments affecting saliva production.

- **Treatment:**

Extensive restorative dental work, including fillings, crowns, or extractions.

Addressing underlying causes like diet or systemic conditions.

Nursing Bottle Caries (Early Childhood Caries):

- **Definition:** A specific type of rampant caries found in young children, often caused by prolonged exposure to sugary liquids from bottles or sippy cups.
- **Causes:**

Frequent and prolonged use of bottles or sippy cups filled with milk, juice, or sugary drinks, especially during naps or bedtime.

Lack of proper oral hygiene in infants and toddlers.

Affected Population: Typically occurs in children under the age of 5.

- **Tooth Involvement:**

Primarily affects the maxillary anterior teeth (upper front teeth), as they are most exposed during sucking.

Posterior teeth can also be affected in advanced cases.

- **Risk Factors:**

Allowing infants to sleep with bottles containing sugary liquids.

Breastfeeding on demand throughout the night without cleaning teeth.

Delayed introduction of proper oral hygiene practices.

- **Treatment:**

Restorative procedures (e.g., crowns, fillings).

Education for parents on feeding practices and oral hygiene.

Preventive measures like fluoride application or sealants.

Comparison of Rampant Caries vs. Nursing Bottle Caries:

Aspect	Rampant Caries	Nursing Bottle Caries
Population	All age groups	Primarily infants and toddlers
Cause	Poor oral hygiene, diet, xerostomia	Prolonged exposure to sugary liquids
Commonly Affected Teeth	Anterior and posterior teeth	Maxillary anterior teeth first
Progression	Rapid and widespread	Starts with front teeth, spreads later
Prevention	Improved oral hygiene, diet changes	Avoid sugary bottles, nighttime cleaning.

Prevention Tips:

- **For Rampant Caries:**
- Maintain regular dental checkups.
- Brush twice daily with fluoride toothpaste.
- Limit sugary and acidic foods/drinks.
- Address underlying health conditions or medications causing dry mouth.
- **For Nursing Bottle Caries:**
- Avoid putting infants to bed with bottles containing sugary liquids.
- Transition to drinking from a cup by 12 months.
- Start cleaning the child's gums and teeth as soon as the first tooth erupts.
- Use fluoride toothpaste appropriate for the child's age.

Both conditions require timely intervention to prevent further complications and maintain oral health.

If you know:

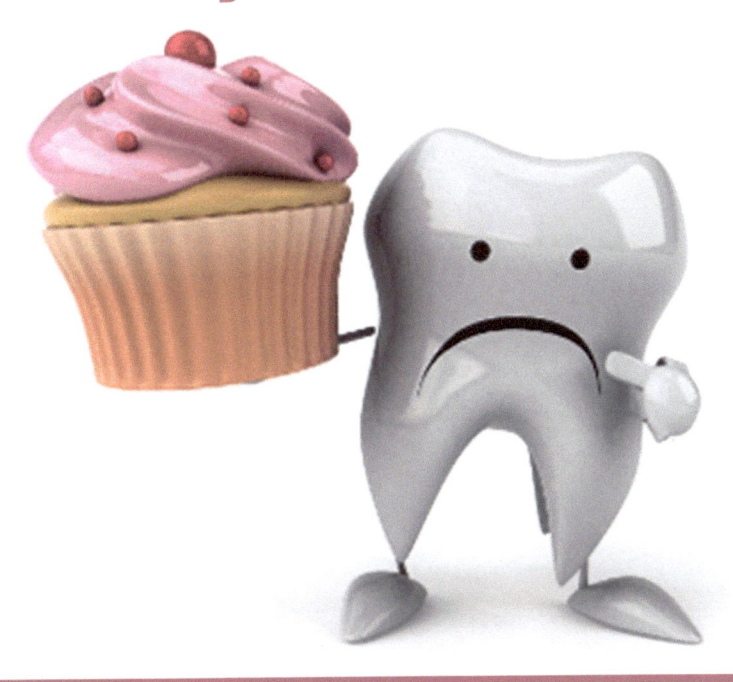

Excessive sugar consumption is a primary contributor to tooth decay, a prevalent dental issue affecting individuals worldwide. The process begins when oral bacteria, notably Streptococcus mutans, metabolize sugars from our diet, producing acids that erode tooth enamel and lead to cavities.

Mechanism of Sugar-Induced Tooth Decay:
1. **Sugar Intake:** Consuming foods and beverages high in sugars introduces fermentable carbohydrates into the mouth.
2. **Bacterial Metabolism:** Oral bacteria, particularly Streptococcus mutans, metabolize these sugars, producing acids as by-products.
3. **Acid Production:** The acids lower the pH in the oral environment, leading to demineralization of the tooth enamel.
4. **Enamel Demineralization:** Prolonged exposure to these acids weakens the enamel, resulting in the formation of cavities.

Preventive Measures:

- **Dietary Modifications:** Limiting the intake of sugary foods and beverages can significantly reduce the risk of tooth decay. Opting for healthier alternatives and being mindful of hidden sugars in processed foods are effective strategies.
- **Oral Hygiene Practices:** Regular brushing with fluoride toothpaste, flossing, and routine dental check-ups help in removing plaque and preventing the acid production that leads to enamel erosion.
- **Public Health Policies:** Implementing measures like sugar taxes on soft drinks has been linked to a reduction in childhood hospital admissions for tooth extractions, indicating a positive impact on dental health.

Understanding the detrimental effects of sugar on dental health underscores the importance of preventive strategies and informed dietary choices to maintain optimal oral hygiene.

Epilogue: A Love Affair with Dentistry

I am Dr. Ajna Abdulrahman, a dentist who has fallen deeply in love with the art and science of teeth, time and time again, through understanding the intricacies of the oral cavity. Dentistry, to me, is not just a profession—it is a passion that has grown and evolved, shaping who I am today.

Like many others, I was once a person of diverse interests—drawn to fields like dance and art. There was even a time when I ventured into the world of makeup artistry, completing a professional course right after earning my honors degree in dentistry. I pursued this out of sheer curiosity, eager to explore and experiment. While I enjoyed the creative fulfilment these ventures offered, they were never my dream. They were distractions, delightful as they were, that took me away from realizing the joy I found in dentistry.

In those early years, I juggled my life between dentistry and cosmetology. Yet, as I delved deeper into both, I found myself constantly drawn back to dentistry. It was dentistry that brought me genuine happiness - a sense of fulfillment that no other field could match. And that's when it struck me: the distractions I was indulging in weren't just hobbies; they were a response to something deeper like underpayment, and a work environment that didn't nurture young professionals in my home country.

There was a time when I worked in a hospital where the challenges were particularly sharp. A senior male doctor, well into his 50s, treated me like a junior, undermining my expertise simply because I was young. Patients often hesitated to trust me, gravitating toward doctors with grey hair, equating age with competence. Some nurses, too, compared me to others, chipping away at my confidence. It felt hopeless at times—being in my early 20s, sitting in moments of despair, wondering if I was truly cut out for this.

But growth comes in the most unexpected ways. Looking back, I see now that these obstacles were not barriers—they were chisels, carving me into a stronger, more resilient version of myself. I realized that those moments of doubt were never about my worth but rather about the world's skewed perceptions. It was in those trying times that I found my self-respect and confidence. I learned that maturity is not tied to age, nor is expertise defined solely by years of experience. Instead, both come from your willingness to learn and grow from every lesson life presents.

Dentistry, I've come to see, is a field of boundless expertise. It is not confined to fixing teeth; it is an intricate blend of science, artistry, and care. It allows you to heal, create, and educate. It is a profession that touches live profoundly, offering both patients and practitioners a sense of transformation.

And that is why I write this: to share not only my journey but also the profound possibilities that dentistry holds for the upcoming generation. Yes, you will face obstacles. Yes, there will be moments when the world seems unkind. But those moments will shape you, refine you, and lead you to a version of yourself you never thought possible. The key is to stay curious, stay humble, and, most importantly, share knowledge. I have always believed that when you spread knowledge with sincerity, you gain far more in return—be it respect, skill, or even happiness. To those reading this, especially young aspiring dentists, know that this is a field where you can find purpose, creativity, and passion.

Dentistry isn't just about teeth—it's about touching lives. And if you're willing to embrace its challenges, it will reward you with the joy of making a difference, one smile at a time.

Thank you for allowing me to share my journey. I hope this book has offered you not only insight but also inspiration. May your journey in dentistry—or wherever your passions take you—be as fulfilling and transformative as mine has been.

With gratitude,
Dr. Ajna Abdulrahman

www.ingramcontent.com/pod-product-compliance
Ingram Content Group UK Ltd.
Pitfield, Milton Keynes, MK11 3LW, UK
UKHW051138240225
455495UK00001B/2